E. Gail Trapp (PhD, MSpSc. [Hons], BSpSc., AssDipAppSc., DipTeach) is a lecturer in Health and Exercise Science at the University of New South Wales. Dr Trapp is an academic exercise physiologist and she has established scientific support for interval training as a means of improving fitness and aiding fat loss. From that she has been instrumental in developing the *LifeSprints* interval training program, which gives time-poor people a 20-minute workout that optimises weight loss.

THE 8 second secret

The scientifically proven method for lasting weight loss

A fitter, firmer you in just 20 minutes a day

Dr Gail Trapp

with recipes and diet information by top Australian dietitian Kate Di Prima

ARENA
ALLEN&UNWIN

Because we have no control over the manner in which this program is used, nor the individuals who use it, you use this exercise program at your own risk. If you have any reason to think that an exercise program may be harmful or injurious to you, seek medical advice before commencing this program.

First published in 2010
Copyright © E. Gail Trapp 2010

Allen & Unwin
83 Alexander Street
Crows Nest NSW 2065
Australia
Phone: (61 2) 8425 0100
Fax: (61 2) 9906 2218
Email: info@allenandunwin.com
Web: www.allenandunwin.com

Cataloguing-in-Publication details are available
from the National Library of Australia

www.librariesaustralia.nla.gov

ISBN: 978 1 74175 687 6 (pbk.)

Photography by Paolo Busato
Text design by Ellie Exarchos
Typeset in Australia by Bookhouse, Sydney
Printed in Australia by Ligare Pty Ltd, Sydney

10 9 8 7 6 5 4 3 2

Contents

Part 3   Slimmer

Part 4   Calmer

How this book can revolutionise your life!

Most people know that exercise, healthy eating and relaxation are good for you. How to find the time to incorporate these in your life in this crazy, time-poor world is the challenge. This book provides easy-to-follow programs to increase your fitness and strength levels in a time-efficient, effective way. All the aerobic and strength-training exercises outlined can be done at home at minimal expense – although an exercise bike is definitely a good investment.

As if that isn't wonderful enough, I also provide a simple 20- to 30-minute relaxation exercise and all the information you need to have the best possible diet. And let's be clear here, that's 'diet' as in an eating plan rather than the excruciating watch-every-morsel-you-eat-in-a-boring-kind-of-way sense of the word.

In a nutshell

Briefly, this is what's inside *The 8-second Secret*.

The *LifeSprints* exercise program outlined in **Part 1: Fitter** has been clinically shown to substantially increase fitness levels at the same time as promoting weight loss. If it doesn't quite do it for you, however, I have suggested others that might, alternatives you can add into the mix to make it just right for you. Remember, though, anything is better than nothing, so a brisk 30-minute walk is always an option if you don't feel up to the more active option.

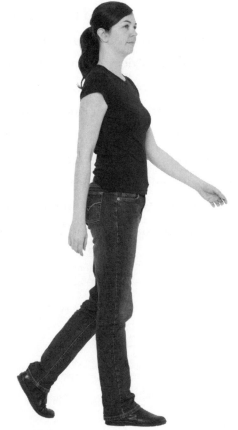

There's overwhelming scientific evidence about the benefits of strength training, particularly as you age. So in **Part 2: Stronger**, provides a range of exercises to work every part of your body, all of which can be done at home without the need for lots of equipment taking over your house. And there are all sorts of suggestions for the program to cater for your needs as there is no point in doing something that doesn't fit your likes and lifestyle as you probably will give up on it if it does. You can pick and choose what works for you.

Recent high-profile scientific studies have shown the health benefits of combining the best of Mediterranean and Asian foods, and this is what I tackle in **Part 3: Slimmer**. As well giving you a list of Med–Asian ingredients to keep in your pantry and fridge, you'll find a number of terrific – and quick-to-prepare – recipes for nutritious, tasty meals in this section prepared by Kate Di Prima. You might be surprised by how simple it is to prepare and eat healthy meals.

Relaxation is not only demonstrably good for your health, it also makes you feel calmer and happier, which is why **Part 4: Calmer** contains a simple relaxation program you can modify and adapt for use in any situation at any time of day. I also include information on how to get a good night's sleep.

How to get started

Start with the idea that you'll put aside half an hour most days doing aerobic exercise or strength training. Okay some days it's just not going to happen, so if you're just not in the mood to exert yourself on any particular day – and let's face it, there will be times when you won't be – then doing the 20-minute relaxation program is a great alternative. You set the program so don't get unduly concerned if you can't do 20–30 minutes every day. Guilt is helpful to no-one.

The best way to approach your planning is to divide your week into the seven days on a grid like this:

Monday	Tuesday	Wednesday	Thursday	Friday	Saturday	Sunday
11 am bike	1 pm strength	9.30 am bike	4 pm strength	10 am bike	7.30 am walk	9.30 pm relaxation

Then all you need to do is write in what you will be able to do that day and perhaps also the time you can do it, as I have done here. Or simply write it into your diary. The idea is to make an appointment with yourself, and to make the effort to keep it.

What I'm providing you with here is an easy and flexible program that you will look forward to doing every day. I understand that there are those days when you'll want to spend any spare half-hour you have just chilling out on the couch watching TV. And there will be occasions when all you'll want is a pizza, a glass of red, and some chocolate to finish. The point is that being naughty on the odd occasion is not an issue. Having pizza (or whatever) regularly is.

TAKE-HOME MESSAGE

Most days you will be able to follow this easy program and it will make a difference to your life. Don't give yourself a hard time if you just can't do something every day – even just a little more than you are doing right now will reap health benefits for you.

Part 1

Fitter

Chapter 1

Benefits of being fit

It's true, and we all know it, those who are physically active lead not only healthier lives, but better quality lives. You can see it in the streets around you. Those who walk tall and freely are more likely to be fitter than those hunched over and tight, and are more likely to smile at you because they feel better within.

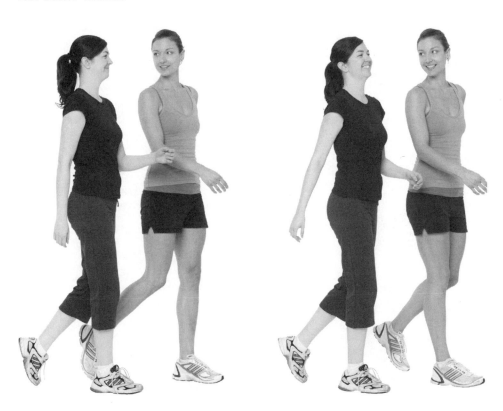

But to be fit doesn't mean pounding the pavement hard for several hours a day. By following our simple *LifeSprints* program you can reap the benefits of aerobic exercise without compromising your lifestyle.

This program will also prevent or alleviate many of the diseases that come from an inactive lifestyle. It is important to understand that these lifestyle diseases not only affect you but your family, friends and colleagues, and there is also a huge financial burden to the community. But what's most important here is: Your life suffers if your health suffers.

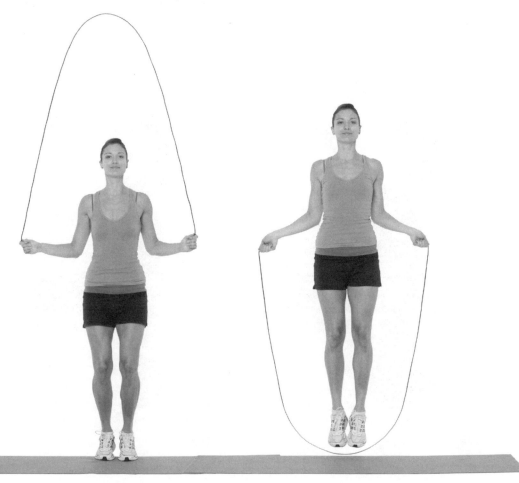

Diseases begone

Regular physical activity prevents you from becoming obese and changes your body composition so you are less fat and more muscular. Apart from the way this makes you feel, being fitter reduces:

- heart disease by lowering blood pressure and total cholesterol in the blood and increasing good cholesterol
- liver complications as it helps avoid the burden of fatty deposits on it
- the risk of a number of cancers, such as breast, prostate and bowel cancer
- the incidence of metabolic syndrome and diabetes
- symptoms of depression
- the development of osteoporosis as bones get stronger with exercise, just like your muscles.

Of course, it isn't as simple as that because your genetic makeup, the food you eat, how you deal with your stress levels and your sleeping habits also have an effect on your general overall wellbeing, but you can *actively* work towards preventing illnesses by keeping yourself fitter.

WHAT IS METABOLIC SYNDROME?

Metabolic syndrome is a collection of disorders that occur together and increase your risk of developing type 2 diabetes, stroke or heart disease. It is sometimes called syndrome X or insulin resistance syndrome. A person is classed as having metabolic syndrome when they have central (abdominal) obesity – excess fat in and around the stomach – plus any two of the following factors:

- raised blood pressure (hypertension)
- high-levels of triglycerides in their blood
- low levels of high-density lipoproteins (HDL) – the 'good' cholesterol – in their blood
- blood glucose levels higher than normal but not high enough to be diagnosed as type 2 diabetes.

How fit are you now?

This is a good time to take stock of yourself. How comfortable are you in your body? Can you walk up stairs without becoming puffed? Do you shy away from activities that require a little bit of extra energy, like playing a running game in the backyard with kids? Be honest with yourself, how fit are you? And then ask yourself, are you getting the most out of your life by not being fitter?

When you follow this fitness program you will be able to quite easily measure your increased energy levels. For example, you'll find early on that you might be able to do only 5 minutes of the program, but within a few weeks you'll be able to do 20, then 30. Give yourself the time you need to build up your fitness level; after all, it's probably taken many years for you to lose it.

Increasing your fitness level will improve your quality of life, health-wise and enjoyment-wise.

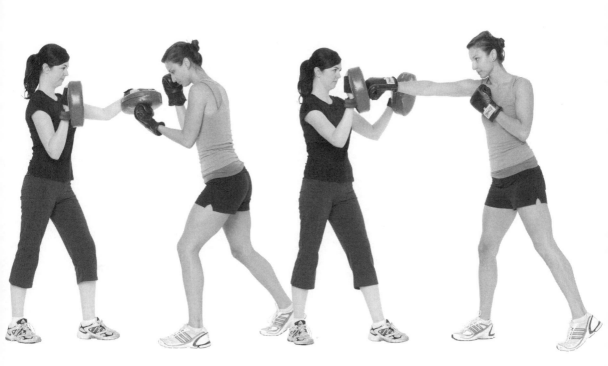

TAKE-HOME MESSAGE

What's important here is that maintaining a healthy body weight and being physically active significantly reduces the chance of acquiring potential life-threatening health problems as well as improves the quality of your life.

Chapter 2

LifeSprints

The *LifeSprints* program came about because, as an academic exercise physiologist, I wanted to study how short-interval, high-intensity sprint training affected fat loss. Traditionally, weight- or fat-loss programs recommend moderate-intensity exercises for so many days a week, for a set period of time (say, for an hour or more, five or more times a week). The rationale is that you burn fat during moderate-intensity exercise, and the more often you do it the more you burn. But many studies showed that this actually leads to little or no fat loss unless you do an awful lot of exercise.

As most people do not have the time or the inclination to engage in five or more hours of exercise a week, we looked into developing a program that would achieve the aims of losing body fat, maintaining or increasing muscle mass, and also be time efficient. That's how my team and I hit upon *LifeSprints*.

What is *LifeSprints*?

LifeSprints is a program where you do a 5-minute warm-up and then 8 seconds of flat-out sprinting and 12 seconds of relative rest. If you are on an exercise bike, during the rest period the pedals simply turn over without much help from you. You repeat this cycle three times a minute for 20 minutes. Afterwards you do a 5-minute cool-down and stretch. All up: 30 minutes.

In our research, we put two groups of women to the test. They came in to see us three times a week for 15 weeks. They would do their 5 minutes of warm-up, then one group would do 20 minutes of *LifeSprints* on an exercise bike and the other group would also exercise on a bike but at a steady, moderate intensity, gradually building up to 40 minutes of exercise at each session. Both groups would then do a 5-minute cool-down and some stretching exercise. The first group committed to one and a half hours per week, the second two and a half hours.

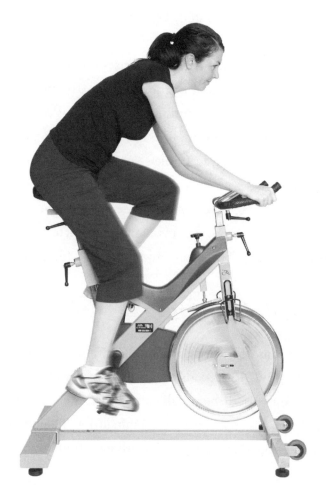

All the women were asked to maintain their usual eating patterns, so that dietary changes would not affect our results. They were also asked not to engage in physical activity other than our sessions.

During the first week, most women in the first group could only do 5 to 10 minutes of the *LifeSprints*; however, by the end of the second week (six exercise sessions) everyone was able to do the full 20 minutes. And, best of all, they loved it. After 15 weeks of training, we retested all the participants. The results were quite a surprise!

The women in the *LifeSprints* group had:

- increased their cardiovascular fitness by 26 per cent
- lost an average of 1.5 kilograms in total body mass – which may not sound like much but some women gained muscle. Some women lost a lot of weight – up to almost 8 kilograms of fat! (We know this was fat loss because the women underwent a DEXA scan, which determines the amount of muscle, bone and fat in your body. It is considered the 'Gold Standard' for assessing body composition.)
- reduced their abdominal fat mass by almost 10 per cent
- recorded a drop in insulin levels of 31 per cent.

The women in the second group:

- increased their cardiovascular fitness by 19 per cent (good, but not quite the 26 per cent the first group achieved)
- on average did not lose weight, and their percentage of body fat increased by 0.6 per cent
- increased their abdominal fat by a tiny amount – 0.1 per cent
- recorded a drop in insulin levels of 9.5 per cent – a definite improvement, but nothing like the improvement shown in the *LifeSprints* group.

Every body is slightly different

Statistics, being statistics, don't provide the individual stories. We found that some of the women in our studies did not lose weight until their blood insulin levels dropped to normal ranges, and sometimes this can take over six weeks of continuous exercise to kick in. Some of the different weight-loss patterns we saw in our groups were:

- steady fat loss – week-by-week a little bit of weight was lost
- delayed effect – participant stayed the same weight for a few weeks then started to lose weight
- very delayed fat loss – participant stayed the same weight for quite a while then suddenly the weight dropped off
- weight loss, plateau, then further weight loss – the participant lost weight initially, then stayed the same weight for a few weeks before losing more weight
- little or no weight loss – weight remained steady, but participant felt better and was a whole lot healthier.

None of these is better than the other. At the end of the day it is what works for you and your body.

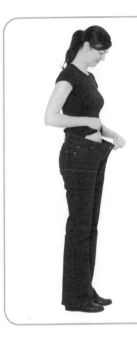

THE JEANS TEST

Assessing fat loss by taking note of your weight on the scales is not a good way to go. As you probably know, muscles can weigh more than fat, so if you are increasing your strength your weight will not necessarily decrease. The 'jeans method' is much more sensible. Put simply, it's the way you feel when you put your jeans or any tight-fitting garment on. As fat is lost and muscle gained through exercise, your body will become trimmer, and this means your clothes will fit better. Take the test!

Getting started

At first, it is important to take things gradually. Big changes do not happen overnight. Be kind to yourself and build up to the full program. If weight loss is your objective, remember it may take a little time for your body to kick in and do that. If you are really serious about losing weight, you need to look at the way you eat. Here, I am talking about enjoying healthy, unprocessed, whole foods as the mainstay of your food intake. Because eating well on a day-to-day basis is so important, there is a whole section of this book devoted to good food that is good for you.

MOTIVATING TIPS

- First and foremost: Make the commitment.
- You might also want to think about doing the program with a friend (or friends) – it's not essential, but it helps.
- Turn on the music – great for inspiration and rhythm.
- Have a clock or other timer that counts the seconds handy. We created a CD (you can order the music online from Music and Motion at www.fitness-essentials.com/index.php?cPath=62) which gives you the in and out cues for your sprinting. While it's not necessary to have this, it does make the timing of sprinting intervals very easy to follow.

TAKE-HOME MESSAGE

If you are interested in improving your fitness and health, then most types of exercise done at a steady pace regularly will do the trick. If, however, you want to lose weight and improve your insulin levels as well as fitness, LifeSprints is a better option. An even better option is to combine LifeSprints with a strength (weight) training program (see Part 2) and adopt a sensible and healthy way of eating (see Part 3).

Chapter 3
Your *LifeSprints* fitness program

Although the *LifeSprints* workout is shorter than the typical aerobic workout it is more intense. So it is important to make sure that this kind of exercise does not exacerbate any injuries or existing medical conditions. You should seek medical advice before you start any exercise program.

LifeSprints was designed as an interval training program on an exercise bike. You do **8 seconds** of flat-out sprinting and then **12 seconds** of relative rest where the pedals are just turned over.

It is also possible to make the sprinting intervals a bit longer. We found that on some machines (such as rowing machines) 12 seconds of sprinting followed by 18 seconds of relative rest worked better. Either interval is fine (the 12/18 may feel a bit harder) so you can set up your workout to suit yourself and the equipment you are using. But avoid making your intervals too long (no more than 20 seconds) because we found that long interval sprinting (say, 24 seconds flat-out and 36 seconds rest) reduced the amount of fat you used to fuel the exercise.

If you don't have an exercise bike or prefer other types of exercise, no problem. Later in the chapter I discuss ways of adapting *LifeSprints* to other methods of exercise.

First, warm up

Make sure you always do a warm-up before you start your *LifeSprints* or the strength exercise program (Part 3), or any exercise for that matter. This is important because gentle activity will:

- warm up your muscles so the muscle contracts more forcefully and relaxes more quickly while exercising, and this enhances both your speed and strength during the workout
- warm up your body temperature, which improves muscle elasticity, reducing the risk of strains and pulls
- activate sweating to prevent your body from overheating
- increase the blood flow to the working muscle, which reduces the risk of muscle stiffness and injury and improves your ability to exercise
- increase the production of various hormones and make more carbohydrates and fatty acids available to increase your energy level
- dilate your blood vessels, which will help blood flow and lower stress on your heart
- improve the mobility of your joints
- prepare you mentally by clearing your mind and increasing your focus – positive imagery during this time can also relax you and build your concentration on the task.

Exercising at high intensity without warming up can cause heart rhythm abnormalities and muscle strains.

All you need to do to warm up is to simply move at a comfortable speed with low resistance, gradually increasing the pace over a 5-minute period. Your warm-up should use the muscles that will be stressed during exercise. So, if you are planning on using an exercise bike, you can just turn the pedals slowly and gradually increase the speed. If you are running or walking, start out slowly and build up your pace. You can also add movements not related to your chosen exercise in the same steady, slow manner; for example swing your arms to help limber up these muscles and increase your flexibility. There is no point in doing static stretching in a warm-up. It does not increase flexibility and it counteracts what you are trying to do by warming up.

Keep in mind that the perfect warm-up is a very individual process but you will find what suits you with practice. Try warming up in various ways, at various intensities until you find what works best for you.

Program options

There are two ways you can ease yourself into the *LifeSprints* program. One option is to start with as little as 5 minutes sprinting/resting, and gradually build this the full 20 minutes. The other is to exercise for the full 30 minutes but start with a long warm-up and cool-down, gradually cutting down the time of the warm-up and cool-down periods and increasing the sprinting/ rest time.

Option 1

WEEK 1

Monday	Tuesday	Wednesday	Thursday	Friday
Warm up 5 min Sprint 5 min Cool down 5 min		Warm up 5 min Sprint 10 min Cool down 5 min		Warm up 5 min Sprint 10 min Cool down 5 min

WEEK 2

Monday	Tuesday	Wednesday	Thursday	Friday
Warm up 5 min Sprint 15 min Cool down 5 min		Warm up 5 min Sprint 15 min Cool down 5 min		Warm up 5 min Sprint 20 min Cool down 5 min

WEEK 3

Monday	Tuesday	Wednesday	Thursday	Friday
Warm up 5 min Sprint 20 min Cool down 5 min		Warm up 5 min Sprint 20 min Cool down 5 min		Warm up 5 min Sprint 20 min Cool down 5 min

Option 2

WEEK 1

Monday	Tuesday	Wednesday	Thursday	Friday
Warm up 10 min Sprint 10 min Cool down 10 min		Warm up 10 min Sprint 10 min Cool down 10 min		Warm up 7.5 min Sprint 15 min Cool down 7.5 min

WEEK 2

Monday	Tuesday	Wednesday	Thursday	Friday
Warm up 7.5 min Sprint 15 min Cool down 7.5 min		Warm up 5 min Sprint 20 min Cool down 5 min		Warm up 5 min Sprint 20 min Cool down 5 min

WEEK 3

Monday	Tuesday	Wednesday	Thursday	Friday
Warm up 5 min Sprint 20 min Cool down 5 min		Warm up 5 min Sprint 20 min Cool down 5 min		Warm up 5 min Sprint 20 min Cool down 5 min

Adjusting your program

Once you have worked your way up to the appropriate timings, then you can start accommodating the program to suit your needs. For instance, if you are time-poor or have more than 20 minutes to give to exercise, simply adjust your program to suit your day or week.

The time-poor person's workout

Monday	Tuesday	Wednesday	Thursday	Friday
Warm up 20 min *LifeSprints* Cool down		Warm up 20 min *LifeSprints* Cool down		Warm up 20 min *LifeSprints* Cool down

For those who have more time

	Mon	Tue	Wed	Thur	Fri	Sat	Sun
am	Warm up 20 min *LifeSprints* Cool down		Warm up 20 min *LifeSprints* Cool down		Warm up 20 min *LifeSprints* Cool down	Walk	Rest
pm	Strength training		40–60 min walk/jog		Strength training	Swim	

The most important thing to bear in mind when adjusting your program is to be realistic. Don't set goals you cannot keep or reach. What you want is a program that fits with your lifestyle and for that to happen it needs to be achievable. And at the same time, you need to aim for a minimum amount of exercise per week in order to gain the benefits. I would recommend you always aim for a minimum of three exercise sessions per week.

Whichever way – you are up and running!

As I mentioned earlier, you need not limit your *LifeSprints* to a bike. You can do *LifeSprints* on a rowing machine, while walking, running, skipping rope, boxing, swimming or during a circuit training session at the gym or in a park.

Exercise bike

Cycling on a stationary bike is an excellent form of exercise. It is non-weight bearing, so it is less stressful on your ankles, knees and hips. Your bike should be set up appropriately so that you minimise any risk of injury:

- adjust saddle height so that your knee is almost straight (but has a slight bend in it) when the pedal is pushed down
- arrange the handle bars so your forearms can easily rest on them
- ideally, the pedals will have grips that work so that you can pull as well as push when cycling. If this isn't the case, use the bike you have anyway and just push.

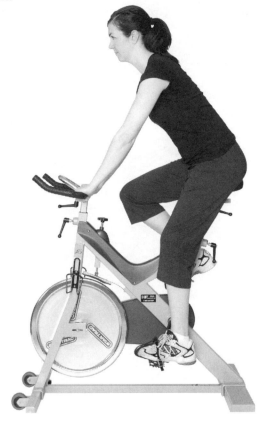

You should be able to turn the pedals at high speed with relative ease. If you feel like you are climbing Mount Everest when doing the sprinting, you have too much resistance on the bike and you need to lower the resistance.

When exercising:

- time your sprint to the music – if you don't have the *LifeSprints* CD, just put on some boppy music that will carry you along and have some sort of timer handy so that you know when to stop and start the sprints
- push and pull the pedals with your hamstrings and quads
- push back slightly with your arms to stabilise your pelvis on the seat.

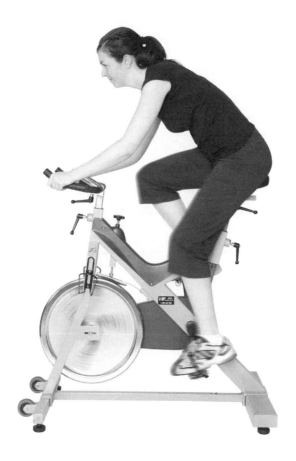

Pushing and pulling with your hamstrings and quadriceps is important because it makes it much easier to attain higher RPMs (revolutions per minute). It also means you use more leg muscle mass and this produces more fat burning. If your bike doesn't allow you to push/pull – just push! It is still a good workout and I don't want you avoiding exercise because you think you haven't got the right bike.

Pushing back slightly with your arms to stabilise your pelvis prevents rocking and bouncing of your pelvis. This avoids unnecessary movement with your upper body and soreness after exercise.

WHAT'S IN A BIKE?

All exercise bikes should have an LCD display showing time, heart rate, calories, speed and distance; have variable resistance levels; have self-balancing pedals with easy adjust straps; and be designed for maximum comfort with level and height adjustments for the seat and multi-position handlebars.

Recumbent exercise bikes are popular because they are comfortable. These bicycles put you in a laid-back, almost reclining position.

Upright exercise bikes provide the feel of a normal street bike, where you sit high and lean forward.

Elliptical cross trainer bikes give you an extra workout as the arms move as well as the legs.

Rowing

Rowing on a stationary rowing machine is an excellent means for doing the *LifeSprints* program. It is non-weight bearing but involves more muscles (upper and lower body) than cycling. A time interval of 12 seconds sprinting and 18 seconds rest is recommended when rowing, as this seems to work best with these types of machines.

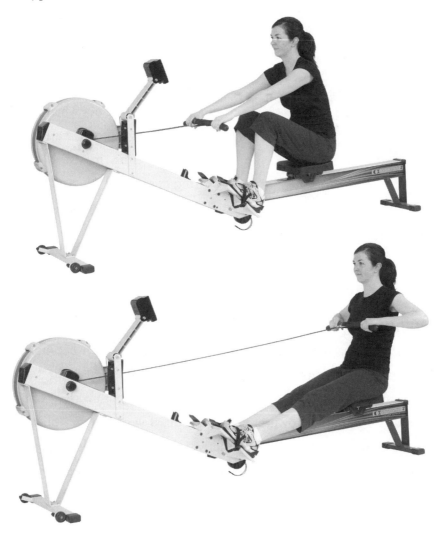

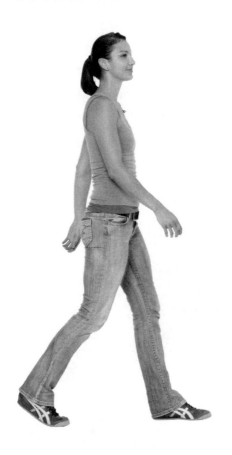

Walking

Sprint walking does utilise the fast twitch fibres in your muscles, but probably not to the same extent as cycling, rowing and running. Nevertheless, it is an excellent form of exercise for those who like to walk. You can use either the standard 8-second sprint and 12-second rest or the 12/18-second interval recommended for rowing. Always ensure you wear appropriate shoes when walking. While walking is not as hard on your limbs as running, it is still a weight-bearing exercise so you need to protect your joints from damage.

Running

Running is an excellent exercise for the *LifeSprints* program because of the easy way you can switch between sprinting and resting. Run fast for 8 seconds and then slow down to almost a walk for 12 seconds, or do the 12/18-time interval as suggested for rowing. Running is hard work on your body, and I would recommend that you leave this activity until you have developed a good fitness base. Like walking, you need appropriate shoes to avoid injury.

Skipping rope

Skipping rope is an exercise you can easily do by yourself or with a partner. You will need a skipping rope (one long enough so you don't trip on it when you skip, but short enough to not be unwieldy) and a suitable surface under foot, as well as appropriate footwear. You could also do the sprint for 12 seconds with an 18-second rest when skipping.

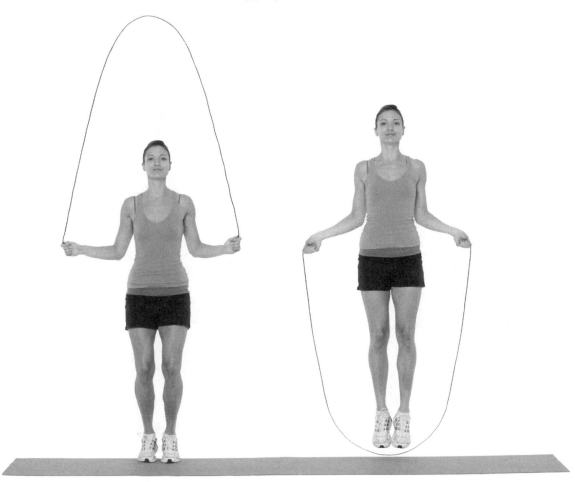

Boxing

Boxing can be done by yourself if you have access to a punching bag or if you shadow box, or with a partner. If you have a boxing partner they can wear foam impact pillows on their hands while you punch fast and continuously into them for 8 seconds, then you rest by moving around the spot shadow boxing (ducking and weaving slowly) for 12 seconds. Once your workout is over, you can do the same for them. Again, this can be done on the 12/18-second intervals.

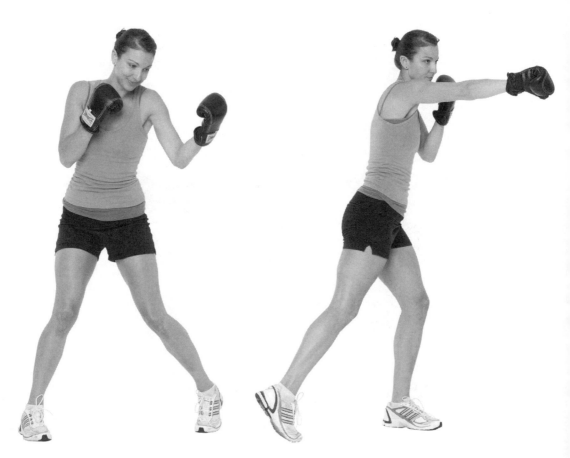

Swimming

LifeSprints can be done in the pool or ocean. The major drawback is obtaining waterproof headphones and music player, and you'll need to be good at counting seconds as you won't have access to a timer. But swimming is an excellent, non-weight-bearing exercise. To do *LifeSprints*, swim freestyle fast for 8 seconds and then slow down to a more leisurely breaststroke for 12 seconds. Or you can sprint for 12 seconds and rest for 18.

Circuit training

LifeSprints circuit training is an excellent form of exercise that you can do by yourself, with a partner, or in a group, although it does take a bit more thought in the planning of it. You can choose a combination of the exercises above. For example, a good whole body workout could include 5 minutes of boxing, 5 minutes of skipping rope, and 5 minutes of cycling, each 5 minutes broken down into the 8/12- or 12/18-second intervals. For the rest portions, in between the sprinting bouts, you could do strength exercises, such as push-ups, dips, crunches, bicep curls, lunges, etc.

Cool down and stretch

Cooling down prevents blood pooling in the extremities of your limbs, such as your hands and feet, which can cause you to faint. Your body needs this time to slowly bring down your temperature and relax your muscles. To cool down you do the opposite of warming up: you gradually slow down the pace over a 5-minute period. On a bike, you decrease the speed a little, then a little more, and then a little more until you are barely turning over the pedals at the end of the 5 minutes and your breathing has returned to near normal.

Remember to always stretch your muscles after you have done your cool-down. Stretching is important because it:

- lengthens and relaxes the muscles you have been using (when you exercise muscles contract)
- helps your body to return to a full resting state
- reduces the likelihood of post-exercise soreness
- reduces the likelihood of postural problems and pain, which tight muscles can create.

You'll need to stretch all the muscles in your body – legs, torso, shoulders, arms and neck. The following stretches will get you started. Keep in mind that the best time to stretch is after exercise because your muscles are still warm and pliable. Stretching a cold muscle can increase the risk of pulls and tears. In order to avoid injury, when stretching remember to:

- be gentle, stretches should be felt but they should not cause pain
- stretch only to the point where you can feel it and hold it there for 6 to 10 seconds
- relax and then repeat the stretch twice more.

Calf stretches

Calf stretches are particularly important to stretch after activities like walking, jogging, running and cycling. The primary function of these muscles is to push off the heel in running and walking. The calf muscles connect to the body's largest tendon, the Achilles.

1. Stand with your hands supported on your knee, with your other leg directly behind, your feet facing forward. You can also push against a wall instead of leaning on your knee.
2. Gently move your knee forward over your toes until you feel a stretch in the back of your calf.
3. Hold and repeat for the other leg.

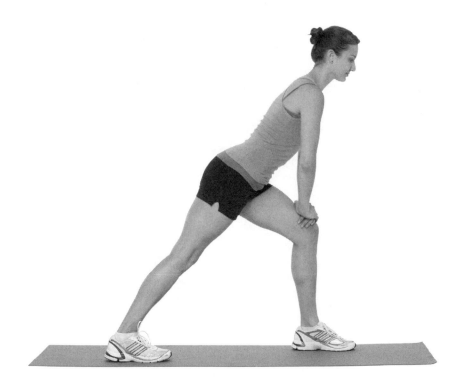

Hamstring stretches

The hamstring muscles run from just below the knee up into the buttocks. They are the muscles that straighten your hips and bend the knees. Tight hamstrings may contribute to lower back pain and cause postural problems.

Stretch 1

1. Begin this stretch by placing one foot in front of the other then lean forward. Support your weight on your bent knee, or use a handrail instead.
2. Flex your foot and push your bottom out until you feel a gentle stretch.
3. Hold and repeat.

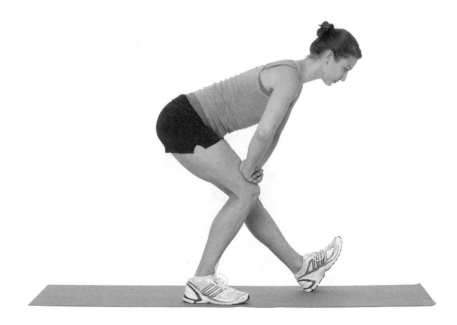

Stretch 2

1. Sit down with one leg straight out in front with knee unlocked and the other leg bent to the side.
2. Lean forward at your hips, keeping your back as straight as possible, and move your hands towards your foot until you feel a stretch in the back of your thigh/knee.
3. Hold and repeat for the other leg.

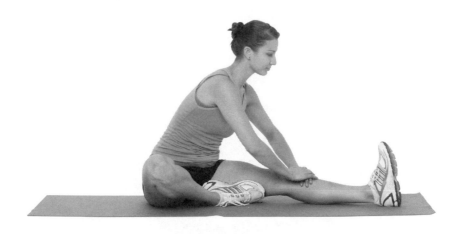

Stretch 3

1. Lie on your back with your legs bent to take the pressure off your back. Make sure your shoulders are relaxed and not bunched up towards your ears.

2. Lift one leg, placing your hands behind your calf or your thigh if you can't reach your calf.

3. Pull your leg towards your chest until you feel a stretch. If your hamstring is very tight, stretch for a short time, move on to the other leg, then come back to a longer stretch of the first leg.

4. Lower your leg to a bent position and repeat with the other leg.

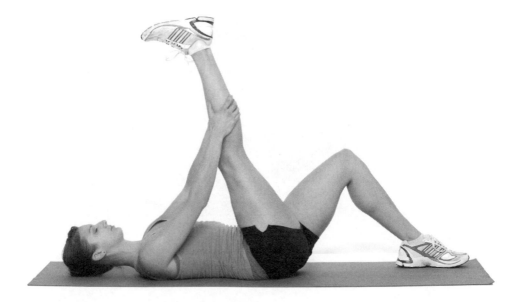

Thigh stretches

Your quadriceps are the big group of muscles on the front of your thigh. Their primary function is to flex your hip and extend your knee, which is very important for walking, running, jumping, climbing and pedalling. Holding in your tummy muscles while you do these will make a more effective stretch.

Stretch 1

1. Stand with one hand touching a wall or stationary object for balance.
2. Grasp your top ankle or forefoot and pull the foot towards your buttocks, keeping your hip straight.
3. Hold and repeat with the other leg.

Stretch 2

1. Lie on your side with your forearm flat on the floor and your spine in a straight line. Make sure you are not straining your neck, and your shoulder is relaxed.
2. Bend your top leg and grab hold of your ankle/foot and pull heel towards your buttocks to feel the stretch in the front of your thigh.
3. Hold, release, and repeat, then roll over and stretch the opposite thigh.

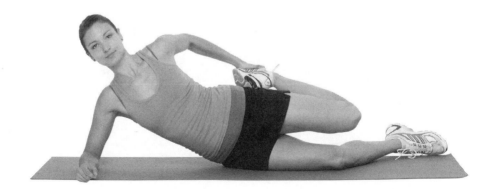

Groin stretches

These stretches are for the adductor muscles of the groin. The main function of the adductors is to pull the legs back towards the midline, a movement termed adduction. During normal walking they are used in pulling the swinging lower limb towards the middle to maintain the body's balance.

Stretch 1

1. Stand with your legs wide apart and feet flat on the ground and facing forward.
2. Shift your body to the left, allowing your left knee to bend until it is over the left foot; you should feel the stretch in the right groin. Raising your arm to stretch your side is optional.
3. Make sure you support your upper body with your hand on your hip.
4. Hold and repeat on the other side.

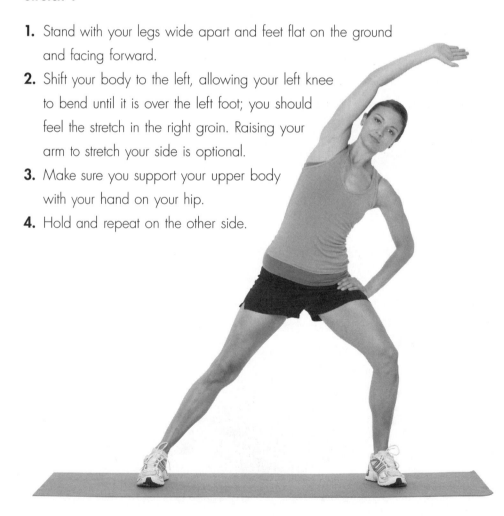

Stretch 2

1. Sit on the floor and bend your knees, pulling the soles of your feet together.
2. Hold your ankles, and push down on your knees with your arms and feel the stretch in the upper, inner leg area.
3. Hold and release, then repeat the stretch.

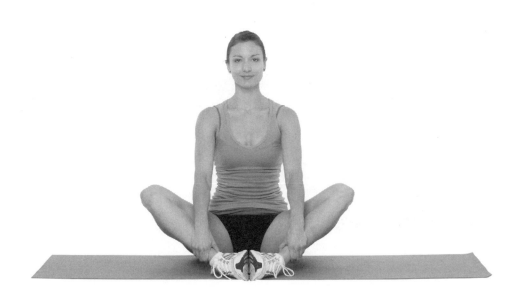

Buttock stretch

The gluteals are three muscles that make up the buttocks. Tight 'glutes' can put pressure on the sciatic nerve and cause pain and also contribute to lower back pain.

Stretch 1

1. Lie on floor or mat, bending your knees. Place one ankle over the opposite knee, place your hands behind that knee and raise the leg ensuring it's at a 90-degree angle.
2. Pull you leg towards your torso.
3. Hold and repeat with opposite leg.

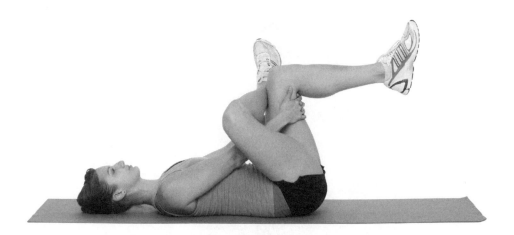

Stretch 2

1. Sit comfortably on the floor with your legs out in front, slightly bend your left knee and place the foot of your right leg so it is resting just to the outside of your left knee.
2. Place your right hand flat on the ground just behind your hips, pushing up to straighten your arm. Place your left arm around your right knee, exert pressure to bring the left side of your body closer to your knee. Keep your back straight.
3. Hold, release, repeat the stretch and then do the opposite side.

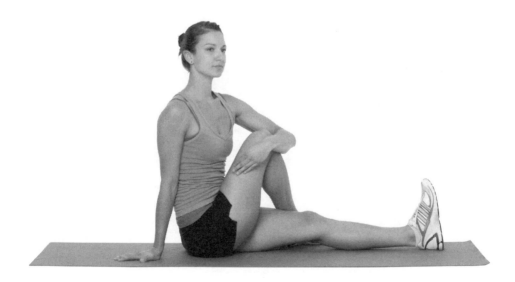

Lower back stretches

This stretch feels particularly nice when you do it, especially if you are carrying any muscular tension.

Stretch 1

1. Start in a kneeling position and stretch your arms high above your head.
2. Bend over, sliding your hands forward and your buttocks back. Make sure your neck is in a neutral position – check your ears are in line with your shoulders.
3. Hold and repeat.

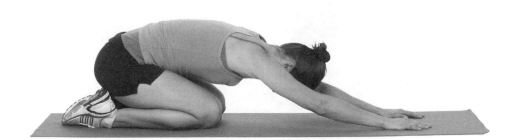

Stretch 2

1. Begin on all fours with your knees under your hips and hands under your shoulders, and your head and neck extended in a straight line.
2. Contract your stomach muscles by pulling your navel to your spine, and round your back upwards as high as you can while you tilt your pelvis inward and drop your head down.
3. Hold, release and repeat the stretch.

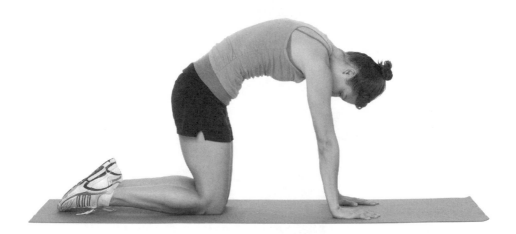

Chest stretches

Tight chest muscles contribute to shoulder problems and bad posture. This is just one of the ways to stretch the chest muscles.

Stretch 1

1. Either standing, kneeling or sitting comfortably, clasp your hands behind your back, with your fingers twined together and elbows straight.
2. Lift your hands out and up behind you as far as possible to feel the stretch in your shoulders and chest.
3. Slowly stand up and release your hands and repeat.

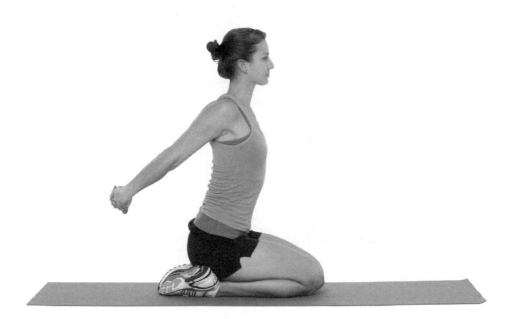

Stretch 2

1. Place your palm, inner elbow, and shoulder of one arm against the wall at chest level.
2. Keeping the arm in contact with the wall, exhale and slowly turn your body around, to feel the stretch in your biceps and pectoral muscles.
3. Repeat, adjusting the hand position either higher or lower on the wall to stretch the multiple biceps and chest muscles, then switch sides.

Side Stretch

A side stretch increases flexibility of your spine and arms, relaxes the muscles and loosens up the torso. It also feels great.

1. Clasp your hands together over your head with your arms slightly bent.
2. Bend to the right at the waist and feel the stretch on the left side of your torso.
3. Make sure you support your upper body with your hand on your hip. Return to the standing position with your hands above your head, and do the same to the left.

43

Arm stretches

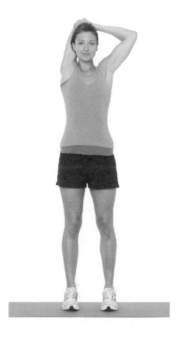

Stretch 1

1. Raise your arm over your head and bend your elbow all the way so your hand is behind your neck.
2. Using your other arm to stabilise your elbow, reach down behind your back and feel the stretch in the back of your arm.
3. Hold and repeat on the other arm.

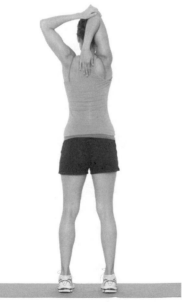

Stretch 2

1. Bring one of your elbows across your body, towards the opposite shoulder.
2. Using your other hand, pull your elbow closer to your shoulder and feel the stretch in the back of the arm.
3. Hold and repeat on the opposite arm.

Neck stretches

When doing these three neck stretches, you can stand or sit, but you need to be comfortable with your shoulders relaxed.

Stretch 1

1. Turn your chin towards your right shoulder as far as is comfortable.
2. Hold, and then repeat to the other side.

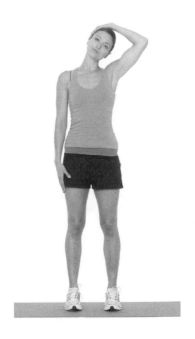

Stretch 2

1. Place one hand over your head and gently pull ear down towards your shoulder, keeping your neck as relaxed as possible. Keep the opposite arm straight and shoulder relaxed, not raised.
2. Hold and release by bringing your head back up, then repeat to the other side.

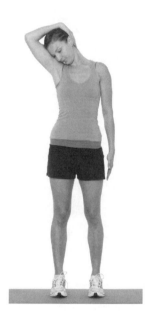

Stretch 3

1. Stand straight with your feet hip-width apart, and your shoulders relaxed.

2. Place one hand over your head and turn your face towards your underarm. You can point your other arm towards your feet for a stronger stretch.

3. Use your hand to gently pull your head down. Hold and repeat on the other side.

TAKE-HOME MESSAGE

Always do a warm-up before you start and a cool-down followed by a stretch after doing *LifeSprints*. You can adapt the *LifeSprints* principles to any exercise you prefer. Simply ensure your equipment is safely and appropriately set up, and that you are wearing the right kind of footwear for the exercise. Once you have a hang of the program, you can easily adjust it to suit your lifestyle.

Part 2
Stronger

Chapter 4
Benefits of being strong

There is a perception that as you age you lose strength. To an extent, that's true because after about 30 years of age you start to lose muscle mass. This loss of muscle mass is one of the reasons you get fatter as you age. Of course, another reason you get fatter as you age is because you become less active! Strength training helps to keep you active and prevent both the muscle loss and fat gain.

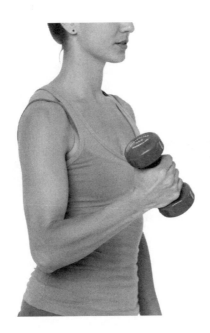

Move it or lose it

One of the major objections women have to engaging in strength training is the concern that they will end up big and muscle bound. That is an unlikely (but not impossible) outcome. To develop big muscles a number of factors need to be present:

- you need to have relatively high levels of the male sex hormone, testosterone – women do produce testosterone but usually at levels that will not cause excessive muscle development
- even if you are male, you need to do a lot of heavy weight training; with light strength training it is unlikely you will develop large muscles
- big muscles are likely to develop only if you have lots of fast twitch muscle fibres.

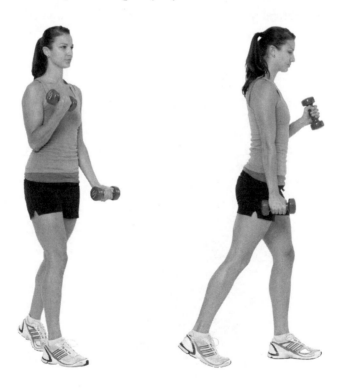

WHAT ARE FAST TWITCH MUSCLE FIBRES?

These are the muscle fibres that tend to bulk up when you train. Young sprinters usually have a high percentage of fast twitch fibres in their muscles as this is what gives them the power they need to run the short distances fast. People with a higher percentage of fast twitch fibres tend to put on muscle bulk more easily than those who have a higher percentage of slow twitch fibres.

If you tend to put on muscle easily when you get active, you probably have a high percentage of these muscle fibres. The only way to find out for sure what your muscle fibre profile is to have a muscle biopsy (take out a chunk of muscle) and have it tested – but this is uncomfortable and messy and completely unnecessary. In any case, unless you are training like a super athlete, it is unlikely to be an issue.

Without a doubt, strength training has been shown to:

- increase the metabolic activity of your muscles
- improve your bone structure and reduce the likelihood of osteoporosis
- strengthen your body so you are less likely to incur injuries and you will also recover more quickly from injuries
- improve your blood sugar levels
- increase overall strength and improve your daily functioning
- help maintain fat loss
- improve your balance.

The loss of muscle mass is one of the potential problems associated with weight loss, particularly in diet-induced weight-loss programs. Some studies have also shown a loss of muscle mass in programs that combined diet and aerobic exercises to induce weight loss. When you lose muscle mass, you lose metabolically active tissue, which in effect means your body is not using as much energy to maintain its basic functioning. Most of the energy your body uses in a day supports these basic physiological processes and when your metabolic rate decreases you use less energy while doing your daily activities.

So, if you continue to eat the same amount and type of food every day, over the long term, you will gain weight. On average people gain about 3.5 kilograms every decade of life which is due to small errors in energy balance caused in part by declining muscle mass. Strength training can help to prevent the loss of muscle mass associated with ageing and weight loss and preserve your resting metabolic rate, thus helping you to prevent long-term or rebound weight gain. Also, we found that *LifeSprints* increased muscle mass in some of the subjects.

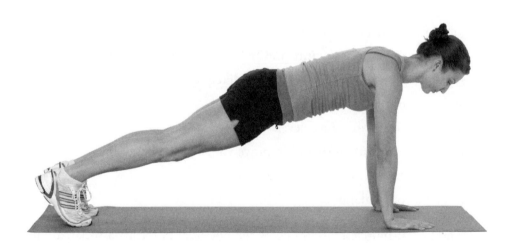

Bones benefit too

Strength training has been shown to induce fat loss without changing total body weight so don't jump on those scales thinking it's all about the numbers. Scales can be deceptive because muscle weighs more than fat so when you lose fat but your muscles get stronger, you may not change total body weight. Taking your measurements is a more accurate way to go, but most importantly you will notice the difference in how you feel and look and how your clothes fit.

Strength training is also essential for strong bones. Bones are like muscle, they respond to appropriate loading by getting bigger and stronger. This is particularly important for preventing osteoporosis and fractures as you age. Not only can it prevent bone loss, but the more bone mass you accumulate when you are younger, the less likely you are to suffer from osteoporosis when you are older. This is especially important for women, who lose bone mass after menopause.

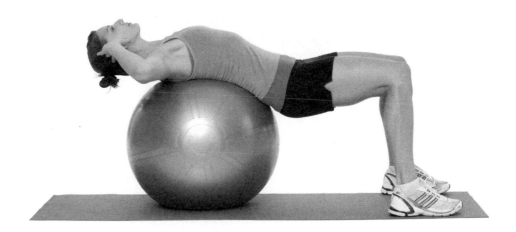

Strong muscles help prevent injury and speed recovery from injury. Strong muscles are better able to withstand internal and external forces that can cause injury. They act as shock absorbers, are more fatigue resistant, and improve coordination and balance.

It is also possible to prevent the development of diabetes with appropriate lifestyle changes. People who have high insulin and/or insulin resistance are considered to be in a pre-diabetic state. Strength training has been shown to improve insulin sensitivity and reduce the levels of fasting insulin, so it is a useful therapy for improving insulin levels and reducing the likelihood of developing diabetes or for managing existing type 2 diabetes.

TAKE-HOME MESSAGE

Engaging in strength training is not likely to give you big muscles. It will, however, make you stronger and more toned so that you feel better and look better. It helps keep your bones healthy and prevents injury, and speeds recovery from injury. Strength training also works towards preventing weight gain and adult on-set diabetes.

Chapter 5

What is strength training?

People think of strength training as something you do in a gym surrounded by big-muscled people who lift really heavy weights. It certainly is something you can do in a gym or health club setting and, if that environment suits you, by all means go there. You may find it useful to go to one of these centres to get tips on weight-training techniques but it is not essential. All the exercises you do in a gym can easily be done in your own home, office or the local park, at a fraction of the cost.

Getting stronger

Strength training – often called weight training – is simply working your muscles against a resistance. That resistance may be your body weight; for example, when you do push-ups, crunches or chin-ups. Strength can also come from lifting weights such as barbells, dumbbells, machine weights, or tins of dog food. Thick rubber bands or tubing also provide a good resistance workout and the bands are easily portable.

The basic principle behind successful strength training is 'progressive overload'. All that means is you regularly adjust the amount of resistance so you are gradually working harder (pushing more weight) as your strength increases. If you do not overload your muscles, there is no need for them to adapt and change, and they stay the same or diminish in capacity.

You can start your strength training program by doing simple things like squats or lunges while waiting for the kettle to boil. Or, do some push-ups and crunches as a part of your cool-down after your *LifeSprints* workout. Get yourself a rubber exercise band to use while you are sitting at your desk or watching television. You can also do a formal strength training program (see the next chapter).

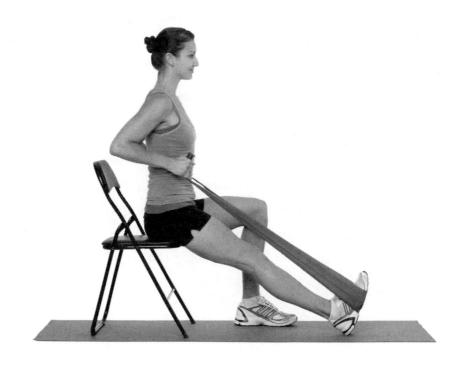

Move, and keep moving

Researchers found that those who engage in set exercise programs often then feel it is okay to reduce their incidental or ambient activity. This means they come home and flop on the couch and watch TV, feeling it's their reward for working out. It is important that you do not engage in the 'I did my workout, so I can reward myself by sitting down with a box of chocolates' type of behaviour. Those who maintain a normal weight or have successfully maintained weight loss are likely to be much more physically active in their day-to-day routines.

It is important to engage in formal physical activity but to also keep up low-level ambient (informal) activity. So reduce your sedentary activity. The evidence that a sedentary lifestyle is one of the main culprits in the rise of obesity and its associated diseases is overwhelming.

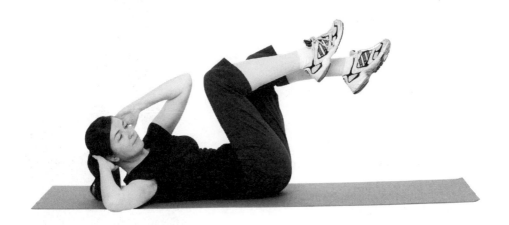

Here are some ways of increasing physical activity:

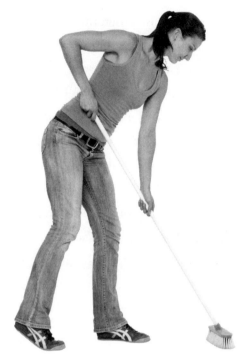

- Get a dog and walk it regularly – it is good for both you and the dog.
- Sweep using a broom instead of vacuuming.
- Chop the vegetables with a knife and chuck your food processor away (or put it in a cupboard).
- Walk up the stairs instead of using the elevator or escalator.

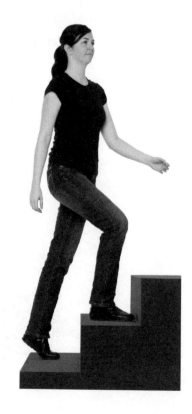

- Stroll to the shops instead of taking the car.
- Take public transport as it will involve walking – and it is good for the environment.
- Take up a hobby so that you don't go home from work and plonk yourself down in front of the TV or the computer.

- Throw away the remote so you have to get up to change the channels, and during ad breaks get up and do something.
- At work, go and speak to your colleagues in person instead of emailing them – it not only increases your activity but it improves your professional relationships and communications.
- Twitch. Move. Tap your feet when sitting. There is evidence that 'twitchy' people are leaner than those who just sit still. Look around you and you will generally find that leaner folk move more and find it harder to sit still.

TAKE-HOME MESSAGE

To build strength you need to work your muscles. Squats, push-ups, chin-ups and lifting weights will build muscle. You can easily incorporate these activities into your day, and it is important to keep moving as much as you can throughout your day.

Chapter 6

Strength-training program

Ideally you should do strength training three times a week, but anything is better than nothing as long as you don't overdo it. I would suggest you try to set aside 20 minutes on the days you are not doing your *LifeSprints* program. Or, if you have the time, do it after you've done your *LifeSprints* workout. As with any exercise, it is important you do not cause injury to yourself. See your doctor if you have doubts about your ability to do these exercises and always wear appropriate footwear and take care with weights.

The program in this chapter uses compound, multi-joint exercises for the simple reason that you get more bang for your buck (more muscles worked in less time). The weight or resistance you use depends on your own strength and the particular exercise you do. For example, you can lift your body weight in a lunge or squat exercise which uses the big muscles in your legs, but you may find that lifting your body weight with your arms (as in a push-up or a chin-up) is nearly impossible – or outright impossible! When starting out, pick a weight that you can lift in a controlled fashion for 12 to 15 times.

Starting program

This program assumes that you are doing your *LifeSprints* on Monday, Wednesday and Friday. However, there is no reason you can't do these exercises during ad breaks while watching TV or after you have done your *LifeSprints* workout. Make sure you do a warm-up before and a cool-down and stretch afterwards. Take it slowly, and then gradually build up your repetitions and the amount of weight you lift.

Tuesday	Thursday	Saturday
10 squats	10 bent over rows	10 knee lifts
10 lunges	10 push-ups on knees	10 step-ups
10 crunches	10 shoulder presses	10 seated rows
10 back extensions	10 side crunches	10 wall push-ups
	10 hip extensions	10 crunches with a twist

Strength-building exercises

These exercises require little equipment. You can buy or borrow dumbbells, exercise bands and extras like fitballs or go to a gym but you can also use ordinary household items, such as cans of food.

It doesn't really matter what order you do the exercises in, but generally you would do the big muscle exercises first. The order in the program provided should give you the idea. Remember to warm up before and cool down and stretch after strengthening exercise (see Chapter 3). Unlike the stretching exercises which are designed to relax your muscles, here you are working towards contracting them so you use them hard, but not so hard as to cause an injury.

The other thing to remember is that you can easily incorporate a lot of these exercises into your every day routine. Do some wall push-ups or squats while you're waiting for the kettle to boil. Do some lunges across the kitchen. Actively lift the groceries (some shoulder presses on the way to the pantry with the dog food cans) – the possibilities are endless. And you may find that your family is so amused by your activities that they actually join in.

Squats

Squats use the big muscles in the legs: quadriceps, hamstrings, glutes and calf muscles. Squats are a great compound, multi-joint exercise but you need to have good technique.

1. Start by standing tall with your feet firmly on the ground, hip-width apart, and weights in your hands.
2. Lower your buttocks as if you are about to sit in a chair, keeping your back straight and tummy muscles tight. Keep your chin up. Do not bend more than 90 degrees at the knees and make sure your knees do not go in front of your toes.
3. Hold for as long as you can, then come back up to standing before repeating the squat.

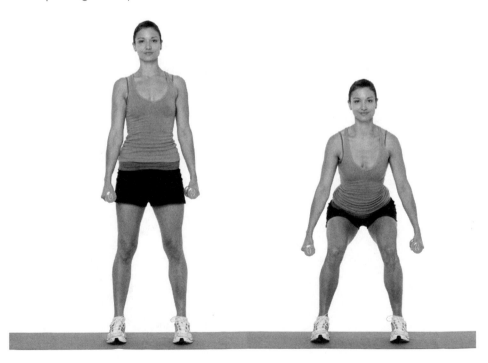

Lunges

Lunges are simply leg squats but with a step forward. The same leg muscles are recruited in this exercise. Brace your tummy muscles and keep your back straight. Don't let your knees get in front of your toes.

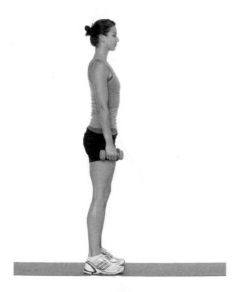

1. Begin the lunge by standing with your legs together and weights firmly in your hands.
2. Take a big step forward and slowly lower your body until your front knee is at a right angle, keeping your knee in line with your middle toe and your feet facing forward.
3. Then step back and repeat for the other leg.

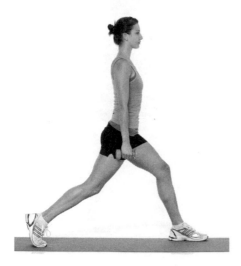

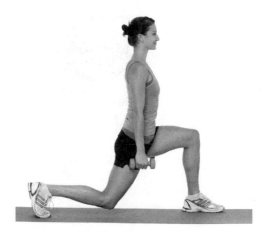

Hip extensions

This exercise works your buttocks and hamstrings and you can start off without the rubber tubing, which gives extra resistance.

1. Support yourself against a chair or other sturdy object and make sure your back is straight.
2. Lift your leg back from the hip, only high enough so your back remains straight. To add resistance, use a rubber band around your ankle as shown. Make sure the object the band is tied to is fixed – you can enlist a friend to sit on a chair as shown.
3. Hold, repeat, and change to the other side.

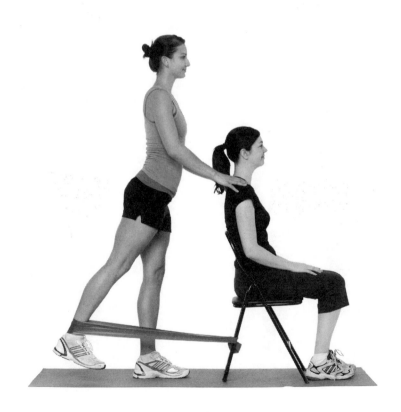

Knee lifts

To twist or not to twist? It doesn't really matter. Twisting uses more muscles but also puts more pressure on your back, so be careful. This exercise works the hip flexors and if you add in the twist, it works your core muscles as well.

1. Stand comfortably with your feet as wide as your hips and raise your arms (you could hold a weight in your hands), but keep your shoulders down.
2. Lift your knee to waist height, twisting your body if you wish.
3. Hold, release and repeat on the other side.

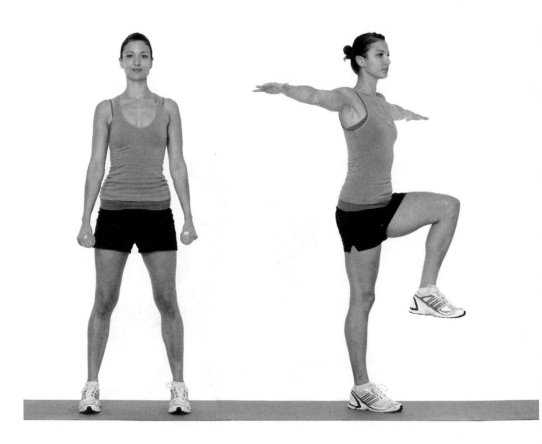

Step-ups

This is a good exercise for strength and an aerobic workout if you do it for 10 minutes or more. It works pretty much all the muscles in your legs and hips.

1. Stand in front of a step, holding onto a handrail for support if needed.
2. Step up with one foot and then the other so that both feet are completely on the step, then step down, returning to your starting position.
3. Repeat, stepping up and down. If you keep repeating this for 10 or more minutes it makes a good aerobic workout.

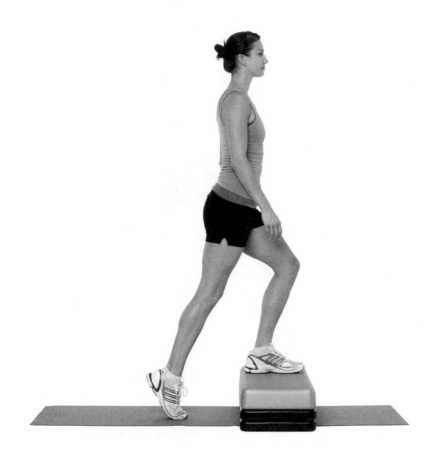

1. Stand in front of a step, feet facing forward.
2. Step up with one foot and then the other so that both feet are completely on the step, then step down, returning to your starting position.
3. Repeat, this time, moving your arms straight up over your head, with your hands pointing upwards as you step up, then lower them as you step down.

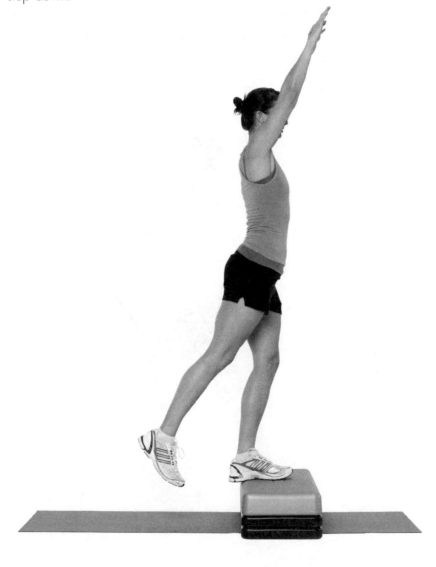

Crunches

Crunches use your abdominal (core) muscles. If lying on the floor is not your thing, do your crunches on a Fit Ball. Just lift your upper body off the floor (don't sit up all the way) and ensure that your hands are supporting your neck, not dragging it up. If either of these options doesn't suit you, stand with your back against a wall and try to push your lower back into the wall by tightening your tummy muscles, relax and repeat.

1. Lie on your back on the floor and bend your knees, placing your hands behind your head or across your chest.
2. Pull your belly button towards your spine and flatten your lower back against the floor before slowly contracting your stomach and bringing your shoulder blades off the floor. Exhale as you come up, keeping your neck straight and chin up.
3. Hold in the upright position, then slowly lower back down but don't relax all the way. Repeat.

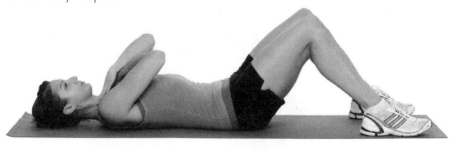

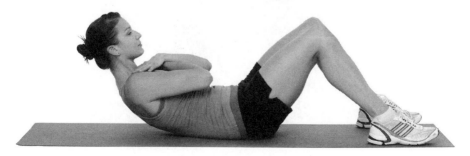

You need to make sure the fit ball won't slip when you use it, so unless you are on carpet, place a non-slip matt beneath you.

1. Carefully place a fit ball between your shoulder blades and hips, with your knees bent, and your feet hip-width apart. Lift your hips so that you are level and not straining your lower back.

2. Place your hands behind your head to support your neck. Make sure you don't pull your neck up, and only rest on your hands.

3. Lift your upper body, your head supported, crunching your stomach muscles as you lift. Keep your thighs firm.

4. Lie back down, and repeat.

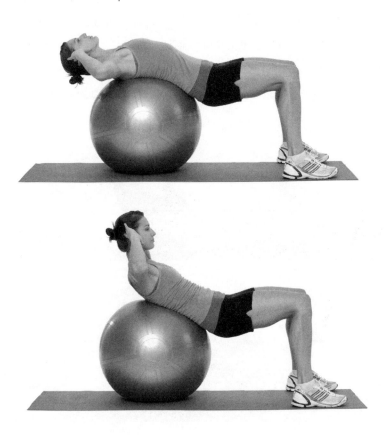

Side crunches

Another core muscle exercise that can also be done on a Swiss Ball.

1. Lie on your back on the floor with your knees up, as in a regular crunch, with your hands behind your head for support.
2. As you lift your upper body twist so that your elbow points towards the opposite knee.
3. Slowly lie back, then repeat to the opposite side.

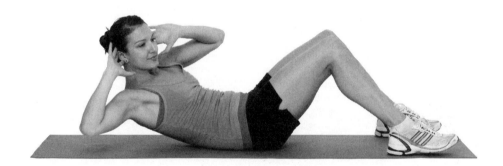

Back Extensions

A great exercise. Your back muscles make up part of the core muscles and weak back extensors (the muscles that straighten your back) have been shown to be a major cause of lower back pain. You can do this exercise on a Swiss Ball as well.

1. Lie face down on a mat and place your hands behind you on your buttocks. Keep your shoulders down.
2. Lift your head off the ground, making sure you only lift your upper body off the floor and you keep your toes on the floor.
3. Hold, then lower your body down again, and repeat.

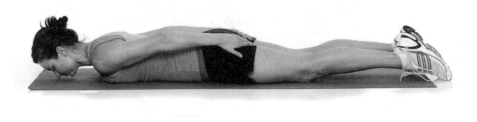

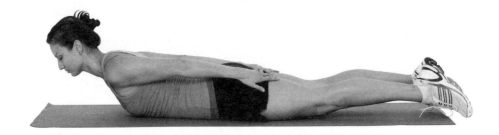

Bent over rows

Rowing exercises use the muscles in your upper back as well as your arms and they are important for preventing poor posture (rounded shoulders).

1. Stand with your knees bent, back straight, and your torso at a 60-degree angle, with weights fully extended in your hand.
2. Bring your hands and the weights straight up to your chest, moving only your arms and contracting your shoulder blades fully.
3. Slowly return to the starting position and repeat.

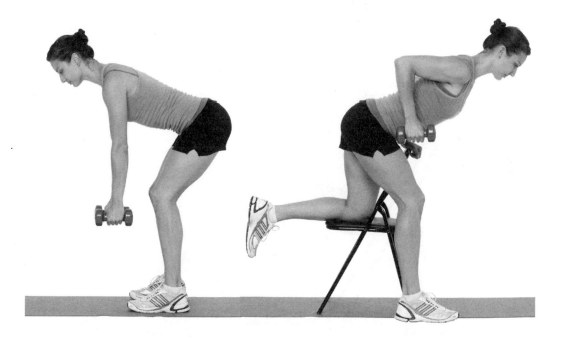

If this position is not for you, try it one-handed kneeling on a bench or chair as shown above so that your body is supported.

75

Seated rows

An essential exercise for the upper back muscles.

1. Sit with your back straight and legs extended out in front (knees slightly bent) with a rubber band around the ball of one foot.

2. Brace your abdominal muscles and pull the rubber band, squeezing your shoulder blades together and release.

3. Repeat.

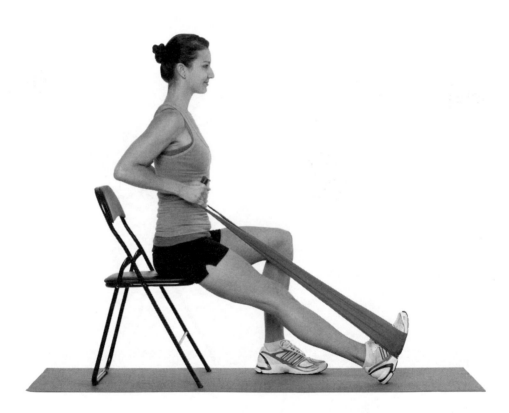

Bicep curl

1. Stand straight, with your feet together and your shoulders relaxed.

2. Place one end of a rubber band under your right foot, and hold the other end with your right hand, fist facing up. Shorten the band by wrapping around your hand if it's too long.

3. Keeping your elbow at your side, pull your hand towards your chest to bend your arm. Release slowly downwards and repeat.

4. Then repeat on the other side.

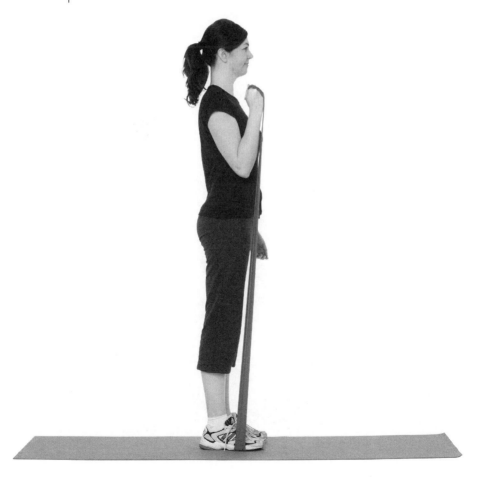

Tricep exercise

1. Sit on a fit ball with your feet firmly on the ground, slightly apart, holding dumbbells in each hand. Brace your abdominal wall muscles to support your back.
2. Lean your chest forward slightly, keeping your back straight and your shoulders relaxed.
3. Slowly push your hand back until your elbow straightens. Lower your arm and repeat.
4. Then repeat with the other arm.

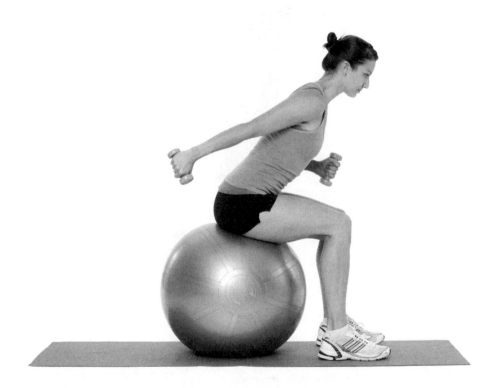

Wall push-ups

Push-ups of any sort use the chest and arm muscles (those flabby triceps!). This is a good place to start with your push-up exercises.

1. Face the wall with your legs hip distance apart and place your palms flat on the wall.
2. Make sure your tummy muscles are braced and your back is straight, then bend your elbows as you would in a push-up.
3. Push back to the starting position and repeat.

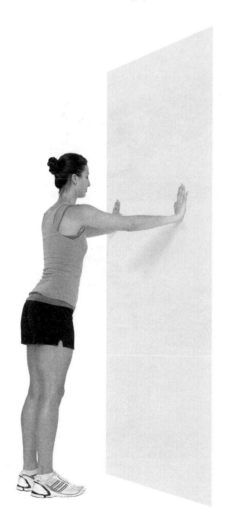 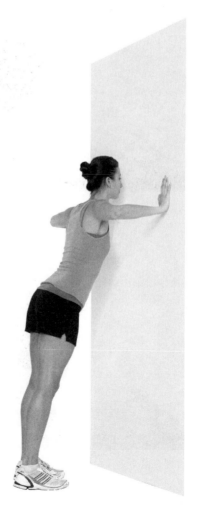

Push-ups on knees

Push-ups are easy and effective for building upper body strength. If your back sags, bend your hips more until your upper body and core strength improves enough so that you can keep your back straight.

1. Kneel on the floor with your knees in line with your hips and your arms under your shoulders.
2. Keeping your back straight, bend your elbows, lowering your body as close to the ground as you can without touching it.
3. Push back up and repeat.

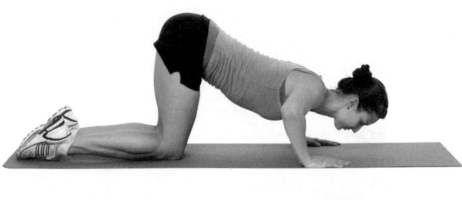

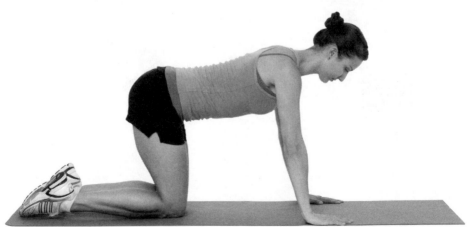

If this exercise is too difficult, try the wall push-up instead.

As you get stronger, you can make this exercise harder by moving your hands further away from your knees and lengthening your body, as shown below.

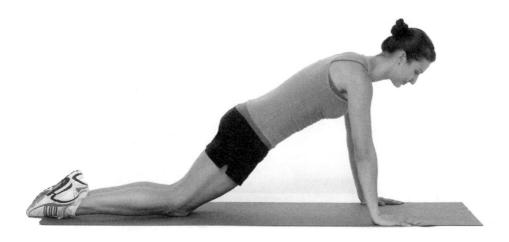

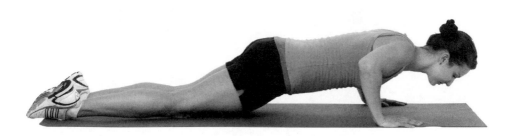

Shoulder presses

This exercise works the shoulder and upper back muscles. You can do this exercise sitting or standing. And, as shown, if you don't have dumbells, you can use cans of food.

1. Sit or stand comfortably, with your feet hip-width apart and weights in your hands with your arms raised and your elbow flexed at about 90 degrees.

2. Keeping your back straight, lift the weights above your head.

3. Bring the weights back down to a starting position and repeat the movement.

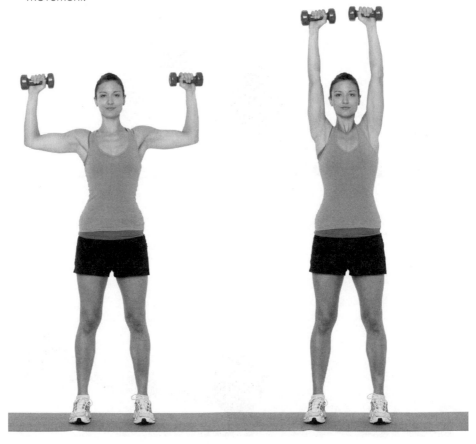

Using cans of food

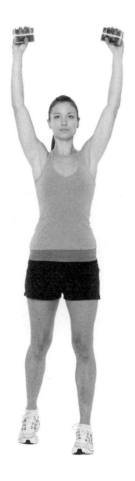

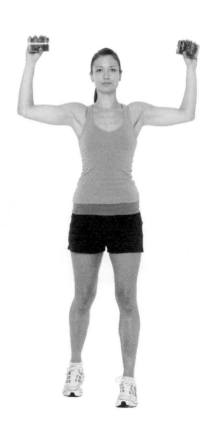

Core strengthening using a fit ball

This exercise works all your core muscles across your trunk. You need to make sure the fit ball won't slip when you use it, so unless you are on carpet, place a non-slip matt beneath you.

1. Lie down flat on the ground with your arms stretched on either side of you and your palms on the ground. Your neck should be in a neutral position so make sure your chin is pointed towards your chest.
2. Place your calves (but not your knees) and your feet on the ball, keeping your feet together.
3. Brace your abdominal muscles, then lift your hips up, using your legs and arms to steady you, until only your head and shoulders are on the ground.
4. Lower your hips so they touch the floor. And repeat.

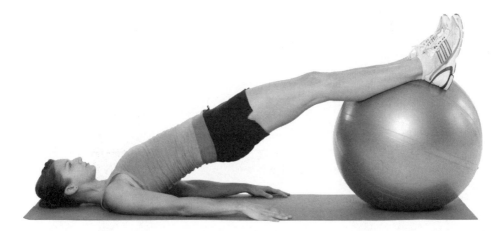

Adapting your program

Start with one set (10 repetitions) of each exercise, then gradually build the number of repetitions up to 15 for each set.

When you can do one set of 15, try doing two sets of 10, building up to two sets of 15 repetitions.

When you can do two sets of 15, do three sets of 10 of each exercise, and so on. When you can do three sets of 15 repetitions of each exercise, add some more weight (use a big can of dog food instead of a little can).

Whatever you use – aim to increase resistance

Once you can do three lots (sets) of 15 repetitions of one exercise, it is time to increase the resistance or work. You can do that by:

- adding extra weight (a 2-kilogram bag of flour instead of a 1-kilogram bag)
- doing the exercise sitting on a Swiss Ball (Fit Ball), which adds a degree of instability to the activity
- find a slightly harder exercise – if you do your push-ups from your knees, try them from your toes
- use a thicker exercise band which will have more resistance
- if you are going to a gym, it's really easy, just add another weight to the stack.

TAKE-HOME MESSAGE

Increasing strength is easily done by incorporating resistance activities into your daily routine. A small amount of effort and you will feel much better and find it easier to do the things you have to do.

Part 3

Slimmer

Chapter 7

Benefits of a healthy body weight and a Med–Asian diet

Kate Di Prima

Frustrated patients trapped on the dieting merry-go-round often lament: 'I assure you that is *all* I eat in a day . . . cutting back has made no difference, in fact I seem to be putting on *more* weight!' Modern weight-loss diets come in all shapes and sizes, from counting kilojoules to restricting whole groups of foods. Even the most disciplined dieter who rigorously keeps a food diary, recording everything they eat, reading every label and restricting so-called 'bad foods', can end up feeling completely deprived and disheartened by a lack of results. To make matters worse, many over-exercise to counterbalance the blowouts in their diet and then feel utterly exhausted.

Welcome to the world of crash dieting, which seems to have become a daily battle for the many people who want to achieve optimal health and weight. Australians spend over $300 million on dieting every year . . . and still the obesity rate rises. Clearly, whatever we're doing is *not* working!

Finding the balance

Busy lifestyles have led to eating on the run, skipping meals, severely restricting kilojoules or – at the other end of the scale – grabbing high-fat, refined convenience foods and neglecting to include fruit and vegetables. This has driven Australia's obesity rate up to the levels seen in the United States and the UK. A typical 'unbalanced' Western diet contains:

- excess kilojoules (also known as energy), which results in weight gain
- excess fat, especially unhealthy saturated fat, increasing rates of heart disease
- not enough fibre, which comes from fruits, vegetables and legumes, leading to bowel complaints
- excess non-core foods, such as soft drinks, cordials, cakes, pastries and fried foods lacking in nutrients essential for the body.

In a nutshell, our eating habits are leading to poor health, ever-increasing weight gain and a huge amount of angst.

To achieve a healthy weight for your height you not only need to balance your intake of food with your output of energy (i.e. the amount of energy you expend with exercise, housework and other movement) but – just as importantly – you need to consume all the macro and micro nutrients required for the body to function properly. The correct weight for your height (measured as body mass index or BMI) is important for overall health and wellbeing because it reduces your risk of heart disease, stroke and diabetes, takes the strain off your skeleton, namely your back, knees, ankles and hips, and makes you feel better, sleep better and generally have more energy. It is *not* about calorie counting and restriction, it is about consuming foods that your body can use.

The concept of achieving a healthy weight is really quite easy; energy in versus energy out. If we consume more than our bodies need, we store it. Yet this principle is eluding more than two-thirds of the Australian adult population because of confusion over exactly what you should be eating and the appropriate serving size, and a lack of incidental and planned exercise.

Given the huge range of conflicting advice from an array of 'experts', it's not surprising that the average person is confused when it comes to their diet. High protein/low carbohydrate diets, high carbohydrate/low-fat diets, low GI, meal replacements, sugar busting, blood types, army diets . . . the list is endless and often misleading, resulting in non-compliance and subsequent weight gain. Some diets are even dangerous, leading to loss of muscle mass, bone degradation or increasing the risk of disease by elevating cholesterol and blood pressure.

Adding to the problem about food choices is confusion over how *much* to eat. Serving sizes are definitely on the increase. Even a basic sandwich has almost doubled in size with foccacia breads, paninis, wraps and rolls becoming so large that many have the equivalent energy of two or three regular sandwiches (a 30-centimetre roll is the equivalent of around five to six pieces of bread!). More of us are dining out too, where large serving sizes are often the norm.

Which brings me to the issue of buying out. The convenience food market has exploded in the last ten years, providing quick and easy options for meals and snacks. While some convenience-food meals may look harmless they can be laden with kilojoules.

To lose weight you need to combine exercise (as discussed in Parts 1 and 2) with a change in your regular eating pattern. Adopting a sensible way of eating and making sure you exercise more will ensure healthy long-term weight loss.

HOW TO EAT WELL

After 18 years as an accredited practising dietitian helping clients lose weight, I have seen most diets come and go or do the rounds under another name. In short there are a couple of tried-and-true principles to help you shed unwanted fat mass.

1. Eat regularly. I recommend every three hours as this allows you a snack in between breakfast and lunch as well as one in the afternoon to get you through to dinner. My clients have had great success when eating three smaller meals and three snacks containing all the necessary nutrients for the day and helping to control their appetite, especially at the next meal. It's important that you eat until you're almost satisfied – don't stuff yourself!

2. Have plenty of water for hydration.

3. Choose good quality protein containing low amounts of saturated fat to ensure the body maintains its muscle mass for metabolic rate. Excellent protein sources include fish, lean poultry, eggs, legumes and small amounts of lean red meat.

4. Steer away from highly refined, empty kilojoule foods and choose grain breads and cereals (bread, pasta and rice are all healthy for you!) and plenty of fruit, vegetables and salads. Full of fibre, these help to empty the bowel and curb the appetite.

5. Move to change the relationship you have with food. If you turn to food for comfort or use it as a reward – or worse as a punishment – you need to work on changing habits and the psychology of eating. Discover how food can nourish and provide long-term enjoyment rather than relying on a quick chocolate fix when you are tired or emotional.

6. Reduce your serving sizes. This may mean getting someone else to plate up your meal so you're not tempted to overfill. Otherwise, simply take a few spoonfuls off your plate and eat a slightly smaller meal.

7. Look at the proportions of different foods on your plate. Lean protein (fish, poultry, eggs, legumes or lean meat) should take up a quarter of your plate, as should slow-release carbohydrates, such as rice, pasta, potato or couscous. This leaves half the plate for vegetables and salad.

What should we be eating?

A vast array of research has found that the traditional diets consumed in the Mediterranean and Asian regions are amongst the healthiest. Both are abundant in grains, vegetables, fruits and legumes, with small amounts of lean meats and dairy. The emphasis is on consuming fish regularly and obtaining healthy unsaturated fats from plants, nuts and fish.

The Med–Asian diet contains foods that are predominantly unrefined, meaning they have had very little or no processing. Examples of these are fruits, vegetables, salads, nuts, seeds, legumes, eggs, fish, poultry and small cuts of lean red meat. This maintains the food's vibrant colours, wonderful aromas and rich tastes. Flavouring meals comes from herbs, spices and oils and using a quick high heat to stir-fry and seal in the goodness or slow-cooking technique to reduce sauces concentrating their natural flavours. I have included my lists of natural flavour enhancers in the pantry staples list in Chapter 8.

Eating with friends and family is traditional to the Med–Asian way of life. Mealtimes are about getting together with your loved ones to enjoy food.

People tend to eat slowly, savouring every mouthful, talking to each other all the while, which can help de-stress. It's all part of nurturing the body and mind in a way that seems to be disappearing in our western lifestyle.

TEN GOOD REASONS TO CHOOSE THE MED–ASIAN CUISINE

1. It is balanced, providing all the necessary macro and micro nutrients for a healthy body, so you have a much better chance of maintaining your weight within the required range.

2. It can add years to your life. In regions such as Greece and Japan where many in the population adhere to this way of eating, their average lifespan is longer than those found in more westernised countries.

3. It is delicious, without all the preservatives and artificial colours and flavours found in cuisines with more refined foods.

4. It promotes moderation and not deprivation, with moderate red wine intake, nuts, seeds and monounsaturated oils that mean you are more likely to stick with your menu plan rather than yo-yo dieting.

5. It contains foods such as fruits, vegetables, grains, nuts and seeds with strong disease-fighting components such as antioxidants and flavinoids, which are important for reducing your risk of different types of cancers and cardiovascular disease.

6. Studies using the basic foods of the Med–Asian diets have been shown to improve the profile of blood fats (namely reducing cholesterol) and decrease the insulin resistance and glucose intolerance seen in patients with type 2 diabetes.

7. Studies using the Med–Asian diets have shown a trend in blood pressure reduction, reducing the risk factors for heart and blood vessel disease. Namely, there is a reduction in the diastolic reading (pressure when the heart is relaxed).

8. It has a low glycaemic index (low GI), which is a measure of how quickly glucose rises in the blood after a meal or snack. Low-GI diets give you more sustained energy, better diabetes control and can help you lose weight by keeping your insulin levels in check.

9. Recent studies in Spain have shown an association between a Mediterranean diet and decreased risks of developing Parkinson's and Alzheimer's disease as well as reducing the incidence of depression.

10. It may have a positive effect on lowering rates of allergies and respiratory problems such as asthma and rhinitis. High levels of omega 3 with anti-inflammatory properties and antioxidants may be the key to these beneficial outcomes.

TAKE-HOME MESSAGE

To achieve optimal health you need to combine good food and make lifestyle changes such as increasing your daily activity and reducing your stress.

Chapter 8

Your Med–Asian pantry and fridge staples

Fresh produce markets and well-stocked grocery stores mean that international cuisines commonly grace the family dinner table. My favourite meal is a super quick chicken stir-fry, my husband loves risotto, my daughter Rosie loves pasta and my son Jack is a sushi fan. These meals are healthy, easy to prepare and cheap, with accessible ingredients from our local shops. Even a quick Mediterranean pizza or Asian omelette is healthier, cheaper and takes less time to prepare than grabbing unhealthy takeaways. These days there is no excuse for eating poorly.

This chapter contains all the essential ingredients you should keep handy to whip up a healthy meal in minutes.

What's in

Try to keep these staples in your pantry.

- **Olive oil** (extra virgin olive oil for salads and dressings). All oils differ in colour, taste and aroma, but the extra virgin olive oil has a deep green colour and rich aroma and I'd recommend using it as the main oil for dressings and salads. Use olive oil for cooking. Full of beneficial monounsaturated fats and antioxidants it is better for you than other fats such as butter and unspecified vegetable oils. It also tastes better and has a longer shelf life. Good quality extra virgin olive oil is a little more expensive as it still contains the protective antioxidant compounds. Beware of olive oil that says 'light' or 'lite'; this just means it's been processed and contains fewer beneficial compounds. In this case 'Lite' means light in colour not light in fat.

- **Fresh garlic.** Recognised as a natural 'cure-all', fresh garlic is full of healthy compounds such as vitamin C, potassium, phosphorus and selenium and the phytochemical Allicin (which gives garlic its characteristic flavour and pungent aroma).

- **Ginger.** Used for centuries as an anti-nauseate, ginger gives a delightful Asian flavour to any dish.

- **Hummus** is a fabulous replacement for butter or margarine on your sandwiches and has the benefit of protein, iron and fibre.

- **Pasta**, brown and/or basmati **rice**, **couscous** and other **grains**. Try to buy good quality, wholegrain, low-GI carbohydrates as these carbohydrates are an essential part of a balanced diet providing long-lasting, slow-release energy. Wholegrain products are a healthier choice than their more refined cousins as they provide fibre to the diet as well as other nutrients like vitamin E. Refined white rice is still nutritious, just think of an apple without its peel. Peeling the skin removes a good source of insoluble fibre and vitamins found just under the skin, however it does not render the fruit unhealthy. Fibre intake is generally poor in westernised countries because we eat more processed breads, grains and cereals and limited legumes, fruits and vegetables. Diets that have adequate fibre are protective against bowel cancer and heart disease and reduce the risk of constipation and common bowel complaints. The Dietitians Association of Australia (DAA) recommends 30 grams of fibre every day. You will note in Chapter 9, there are a number of recipes containing beans and chick peas, which are full of fibre, plant proteins and slow-release carbohydrates that should be included more regularly in our diets.

- **Baby potatoes.** Old potatoes have a higher GI than baby (or Pontiac) potatoes.
- **Fresh fruit and vegetables.** Learn to have a love affair with fruits, vegetables and salads as they are high in fibre, vitamins, minerals and antioxidants. It's great if you can eat two portions of fruit (one serve is about the size of your fist) and five servings of vegetables a day (a serve is ½ cup of cooked vegetables or 1 cup of fresh salad leaves). Remember the more roughage the better.
- **Buy in season.** Choose fruit and vegetables that are in season as they are in more plentiful supply, taste better and are cheaper. Products that travel halfway around the country – or the world – or have been stored in the dark for months on end just don't taste or look as good. There is also the environmental cost of packaging and transporting these products.
- **Dried fruit and raw, unsalted nuts** such as almonds and walnuts.
- **Berries.** Not only do berries taste fabulous, they are full of antioxidants and flavinoids that are very good for you.
- **Fish.** All fish and seafood is healthy, containing mainly unsaturated fat, which is good for the heart. The cooking method is essential in maintaining a healthy fish meal – i.e. avoid battering, deep-frying and crumbing. Choosing oily fish like salmon and sardines provides high levels of the essential omega 3 fats which have been shown to have wide-ranging effects on the healthy functioning of your brain, including susceptibility to depression. The DAA recommends three servings a week (a serve being

80 to 120 grams). If you find fish unpalatable, supplement with fish oil capsules or use flaxseed oil.

- **Poultry.** If you are trying to lose weight, avoid the skin as this is where most of the unhealthy saturated fat lies. Substituting poultry and small cuts (around 65 to 100 grams) of cooked lean red meat three to four times a week is a healthier option and mimics that of the traditional diets found in the Med–Asian regions.

- **Fresh herbs.** Buy, or even better grow, your own fresh herbs, as most do well in pots and are pretty hardy in the Australian climate. Herbs are full of antioxidants and intense flavours, adding taste and texture to your food without adding kilojoules and eliminating the need for large amounts of salt. A useful herb garden should contain parsley, basil, coriander, lemongrass, mint, sage, marjoram, thyme and oregano.

- **Fresh ground pepper spices and onions** (mature, red, brown or spring). Used to season your food instead of salt – a main contributor in elevated blood pressure.

- **Fresh lemons, limes, rice wine vinegar and balsamic vinegar.** Keep on hand for use in dressings, as flavouring or instant sauces.

- **Good-quality curry paste.** If you are serious about your curries you can make your own curry blends from fresh spices and olive oil. But if time is of the essence you can always find ready-prepared pastes in the supermarket. Buying pre-prepared sauces (as opposed to pastes) is not recommended as they are extremely high in fat with some having 'gee' and 'cream' as one of the main ingredients.

- **Low-fat coconut milk.** It tastes as good as the coconut cream and has less fat. Better still, you can use a combination of coconut essence and skim evaporated milk – virtually fat free.

- **Canned fish.** Salmon, sardines and tuna packed in spring water, olive oil or canola oil. Tuna and salmon are naturally oily fish so they don't absorb much of the oil stored in the tin.

- **Capers and caper berries.** These little beauties pack a flavour punch and are a great addition to pasta and salads.

- **Parmesan, Pecorino and Romano cheese.** These hard cheeses are around 30 per cent fat (high in saturated) and sodium; however, you only need a small amount, grated or shaved, to add an amazing flavour to any Mediterranean recipe. Remember, good quality will take any ordinary dish to new culinary heights. Use sparingly and enjoy.

- **Low-fat dairy products.** Skim milk and yoghurt are not common in many Asian dishes but appear regularly in many Greek and Italian recipes. Greek-style yoghurt is a great substitute for cream in both sweet and savoury dishes – adding calcium, protein and healthy bacteria (known as probiotics) to the gut. Skim milk is also handy to make healthy sauces for pasta dishes such as lasagne, cannelloni or creamy spaghetti dishes. Ready-to-eat fruit yoghurt is a healthy snack but you need to be careful of the sugar content. Read the label or, better still, add your own fresh fruit to plain skim Greek yoghurt.

- **Canned chickpeas, cannellini beans** and ready-to-use **legumes** such as red or brown lentils. These are a valuable source of slow-release carbohydrates and protein as well as providing high amounts of soluble fibre and iron. These incredibly convenient ingredients are the basis to many fabulous quick and easy recipes. They are a great substitute for animal proteins and provide little or no artery-clogging saturated fat.

- **Tomatoes.** Next to olive oil, tomatoes are the second most staple ingredient in the Mediterranean diet, and are also popular in Southeast Asian and Indian cuisines. The pigment that gives tomatoes their red colour – which is called lycopene – is a powerful antioxidant that is particularly effective in reducing the risk of prostate, lung and stomach cancers.

- **Low-sodium tomato paste in sachets.** Tomato paste gives tomato-based dishes a more intense flavour while helping to thicken the dish.
- Jars of pitted **olives.** Eat whole, use as garnish, add to salads or crush into a tapenade and use as dip. Olives are high in good fats and salt so eat in small amounts.
- **Salad leaves.** I like baby mesculin (mixed leaves) as it gives you a variety of leaves including baby spinach, rocket and radicchio for a side salad as an addition to any meal. Just add a few sprouts and a drizzle of sesame or olive oil and balsamic vinegar.
- **Asian greens.** Bok choy or Gai lum are members of the brassica vegetable group that also includes broccoli, cauliflower, brussel sprouts and cabbage. They are high in fibre, antioxidants and iron.
- **Sauces and marinades.** Soy sauce (comes in low-salt variety); oyster sauce and fish sauce are essential ingredients in any Asian stir-fry or marinade. These sauces are high in salt, however, so you only need a few splashes to flavour any dish. Look for reduced-salt varieties if blood pressure is a concern.
- **Chilli.** Fresh chilli packs a punch in any stir-fry or sauce (the small red chilli seeds are the most potent, so be careful when you prepare them). Sweet chilli is milder on the palate and gives a delicate flavour to fish meals and salads. It has no fat and very few kilojoules.
- **Bean sprouts.** Mung bean sprouts are an excellent source of vitamin C and iron and add a nutty crisp flavour to salads and stir-fries.
- **Asian mushrooms.** Enokitake, shiitake and oyster mushrooms are typical in most Asian recipes, adding a wonderful texture as well as the healthy properties of vitamin B and iron.

- **Tofu or bean curd.** Gradually increasing in popularity is the creamy texture of tofu. Made from soy beans, it is high in protein, iron and phytooestrogens and contains polyunsaturated fat with little or no saturated fat. Tofu can be substituted in recipes that call for meat, chicken or fish and if added in the last few minutes of cooking, it will hold its form. Tofu also comes in a pourable form to be used in sauces.
- **Hokkien/soba/udon noodles.** Eaten for centuries as an alternative to rice in the Asian diet, and very popular in noodle soups from countries such as Japan and China. Made from buckwheat and wheat flour, they are an excellent source of B vitamins, niacin and thiamine and a source of protein and fibre.

What's out

Try to limit the use of – or find an alternative to – the following

- **Salt.** We use a lot of salt in the western diet, not only as flavouring in cooking but also as a preservative in packaged foods. High levels of salt in the diet increase the risk of high blood pressure, putting the heart under stress. To cut down on the amount of salt in your diet, learn to enjoy the natural taste of food. Don't add salt at the dinner table and use alternative flavourings in your cooking. Use lemon or lime juice, garlic, ginger, onions, vinegar, herbs and spices to flavour your food. Most salt in our diets comes from processed foods, such as breads, chips, crackers, processed deli meats and cheeses. Many Australians have started to use iodised salt due to the lack of iodine present in our soils, however FSANZ (food standards Australia and New Zealand) has recently authorised the addition of iodine to all milled flour in Australia, eliminating the use for excess salt. Rock salt, vegetable salt and sea salt are still all salt! Read the nutritional panels on food. Low salt is less than 120 milligrams of sodium per serve.

- **Refined sugar.** This is so unnecessary in the amounts consumed in the western diet. Natural sugars found in fruits, vegetables and slow-release carbohydrates such as pastas and grains provide all the sugar the body needs. Refined sugar provides empty kilojoules, causes abnormal elevations in insulin, promotes tooth decay, and offers no nourishment. Instead of eating sugary desserts or snacks, have a piece of fresh or dried fruit or an occasional small piece of dark chocolate to finish off a meal.

- **Butter.** Replace butter with olive oil, sesame oil or olive oil spreads in recipes that call for butter. Some recipes may taste slightly different or have a different texture. Use hummus, avocado or pickles, mustard or chutney as a spread on your sandwiches instead of butter.

- Reduce your consumption of **fatty cuts of red meat**. Choose good-quality lean cuts of lamb and beef when you do use them. The Dietitians Association of Australia recommends consuming lean red meat three to four times per week in serving sizes of 65 to 100 grams, which is less than The American Institute for Cancer Research's recommendation of an upper limit of 18 ounces (approximately 500 grams) of red meat per week. One hundred grams is about the size of the palm of your hand, so a maximum of three to four servings this size should be consumed per week. There is no suggestion that red meat should be completely eliminated from the diet as it provides essential nutrients such as zinc and iron. However, in population studies where large volumes of fatty red meats are consumed there are higher risks of coronary heart disease and morbidity. Research into these diets also reveals consumption of processed meats such as salami, bacon and ham. These should also be limited due to their fat and salt content and the presence of preservative 250, known as Nitrate, which has been implicated in increasing the risk of certain cancers.

- **Biscuits** (sweet and savoury), **cakes, cookies, pastries**, pies, some muesli and breakfast bars, **snack foods** like crisps and chips, lollies and **most chocolate**. These are all non-core foods that should make up a very small portion of your diet due to their non-nutritive state. When you buy savoury biscuits, buy wholegrain, low-fat and low-salt varieties. When you buy chocolate, try to make it good quality, 70 per cent cocoa or greater, dark chocolate (and have small quantities). When you want a snack, go for a piece of fruit, a small handful of nuts, dried fruit or seeds or chop carrot, celery or red capsicum into strip for dipping into hummus, beetroot or avocado dips.

> ### TAKE-HOME MESSAGE
> I've said it before, and will say it again: To maximise the health benefits of your diet, try to choose fresh produce and avoid refined foods. Prepare it yourself so you know all ingredients. However, if it comes in a package, read the nutrition panel and choose the healthiest option. You have one body – treat it with respect.

Chapter 9

Med–Asian recipes

Breakfast

Breakfast is one of the most important meals of the day – so make it count. A piece of toast with jam just doesn't have the sustaining energy or nutrients to get you through to mid morning. Take an extra few minutes to prepare something that looks good, tastes sensational and sets you up to make healthy choices for the rest of the day. People who skip breakfast are more likely to choose unhealthy fat- and salt-laden foods at their next meal. If you are strapped for time have some fresh fruit, yoghurt and a sprinkle of nuts and seeds. The following breakfast recipes are quick and easy and can be prepared the night before if time is of the essence.

Bircher muesli

40 g natural muesli (½ cup)
½ cup no added sugar apple or cranberry juice
100 g low-fat blueberry yoghurt

1. Place muesli and juice in bowl and soak overnight.
2. Add yoghurt and serve immediately.
   Serves 1

Breakfast bruschetta

2 slices breadstick (50 g)
1 tbsp pesto (see recipe)
40 g proscuitto (optional)
20 g semi-dried or fresh tomatoes
basil leaves

1. Toast the breadstick pieces.
2. Spread ½ tablespoon of pesto on each slice.
3. Arrange proscuitto, tomatoes and basil on top and serve immediately.
   Serves 1

Pesto, basil and sun-dried tomato take a little while to break down, so even if you choose a white breadstick, this is a low-GI meal.

Scrambled eggs with rocket and Roma tomatoes

2 eggs, beaten
1 tbsp skim milk
pinch salt
1 cup baby spinach and rocket leaves
1 Roma tomato
1 wholemeal English muffin, cut in half and toasted

This dish works fabulously on a barbecue hot plate.

1. Beat eggs with milk and salt. Pour into a non-stick pan and with a plastic spoon drag in the sides of egg mixture as it starts to set (this scrambles the egg). Remove from the pan and set aside.
2. Place greens in the pan until they wilt (takes a few seconds) and lightly grill the tomato, about 2 minutes.
3. Place wilted greens and eggs on toasted muffin and serve with tomato on the side.

Serves 1

Savoury spinach and feta muffins

2¼ cups self-raising flour
1 tbsp raw sugar
20 g olive oil
1 cup chopped baby spinach
200 g low-fat feta cheese, chopped
1 egg, beaten
1 cup skim milk
½ cup grated parmesan

1. In a mixing bowl combine flour and sugar and fold in oil. Add spinach and feta.
2. Beat the egg and milk together and add to the flour mixture. Mix well.
3. Place even amounts into a 12-hole muffin tin and sprinkle with parmesan.
4. Bake at 190°C for 20 minutes (until muffins spring back on touching).
   Makes 12; serves 6

Blueberry muffins

4 cups plain flour
1 cup good quality muesli
4 tsp baking powder
¼–½ cup raw sugar
1 tsp salt
1 punnet blueberries
4 eggs
500 ml low-fat or skim milk
2 tbsp coconut oil (or butter)

1. Preheat the oven to 200°C.
2. Mix together the flour, muesli, baking powder, sugar and salt in a large bowl. Add the fruit pieces and gently mix.
3. In a separate bowl, beat the eggs then add the milk. Melt coconut oil for a few seconds in a microwave and mix in with the eggs and milk. Add to the dry ingredients and mix until just combined. If the mixture is too dry, add a bit more milk; it should not be runny though. Do not over-mix or your muffins will be tough. Lumps of flour in the mix are fine.
4. Spoon into lightly greased muffin tins and bake for about 20 minutes, until risen and brown on top.
5. Remove from the tins when cooked and cool on a cake rack. Eat there and then or put in an airtight container and freeze.
   Makes 12 muffins

Ricotta corncakes with avocado relish

1 cup wholemeal self-raising flour
2 eggs
½ cup skim milk
125 g low-fat ricotta cheese
310 g can corn kernels
2 tbsp grated parmesan
pinch salt and pepper

1. Place flour in a bowl.
2. Combine eggs, milk and ricotta cheese until smooth and add to the flour. Mix well. Add corn, parmesan, and salt and pepper and mix well.
3. Drop large spoonfuls into a non-stick pan and spread the mixture out slightly until it forms a circle.
4. Dry fry until golden on both sides.
   Makes 10; serves 5

Avocado relish

1 avocado chopped into chunks
1 tbsp lime juice
¼ red onion chopped
1 tsp olive oil
pinch salt and black pepper

1. Mix all the ingredients together well.
2. Serve as a garnish to your breakfast dishes or on top of toast.

Lunch or light meals

For many people who live in the Med–Asian region their main meal is enjoyed in the middle of the day, leaving the lighter meal for the evening. This can be popular for Australians in winter but most of us still enjoy having their main meal at the end of the day. You should try to set aside time for a lighter meal during the day and not eat on the run or, worse, skip it all together. Enjoy the following lighter meals for your lunch or evening meal.

Sushi – avocado and Atlantic salmon

1 tbsp sushi vinegar
2 cups cooked short grain rice, cooled
4 sheets seaweed (nori sheets), softened with water
150 g Atlantic salmon
40 g avocado
wasabi (optional)

1. Pour vinegar over the cooked cold rice and mix thoroughly.
2. Place seaweed sheets shiny side down and spread each one with a thin, even layer of rice (about ½ cup each), leaving 3 centimetres along one edge free of rice.
3. Divide the salmon and avocado into four portions and place in a line about 3 centimetres in along the edge opposite the side free of rice. Spread a thin strip of wasabi down the length of the seaweed.
4. Gently roll the whole sheet into a pipe, starting from the end with the filling, and using the edge without filling to seal.
5. Slice the roll with a wet knife to create smaller rolls and serve with soy and fresh ginger.
   Serves 2

An alternative filling is chilli tuna. Mix a 150-gram tin of tuna in springwater with 1 tablespoon of light mayonnaise and 1 teaspoon of mild chilli. Divide into four portions and make as above.

Vietnamese prawn rolls

12 rice paper rounds (120 g)
1 cup grated carrot
100 g snow peas, sliced
1 cup bean sprouts
30 g rice vermicelli, soaked in boiling water, cooled and drained
2 tbsp chopped coriander
2 tbsp chopped fresh mint
400 g (approx 24) cooked prawns, shelled

Dipping sauce

1 tbsp caster sugar
¼ cup hot water
1 clove garlic
¼ cup lime juice
2 tbsp fish sauce
1 small fresh chilli, finely sliced (optional)
1 tbsp chopped fresh coriander

1. Dip the rice paper in hot water until it softens.
2. Combine all the ingredients in a bowl and mix together.
3. Place 2 tablespoons of the mix and 2 prawns on the lower half of each rice paper and roll firmly into a spring roll shape.
4. To make the dipping sauce, add sugar and hot water in a bowl and stir until sugar is dissolved. Add the remaining ingredients and combine well.
   Makes 12; serves 3

Zucchini and corn fritters

400 g peeled potatoes
500 g zucchini
2 fresh corn cobs
1 tbsp fresh thyme or coriander
½ cup plain flour
2 eggs, lightly beaten
olive oil
1 small Lebanese cucumber
1 small carton low-fat tzatziki
1 bunch rocket leaves
4–8 smoked salmon slices

1. Put potato and zucchini in a food processor and coarsely grate. Transfer to a colander and squeeze out the excess moisture. Put in a large bowl.
2. Cut the corn kernels from the cobs and add to the potato mixture along with the fresh herbs, flour and eggs. Mix well.
3. Heat a little olive oil in a non-stick pan and add spoonfuls of the potato mixture to make small fritters. Use an egg slice to flatten slightly. Cook for 4 to 5 minutes on each side until golden brown. Transfer to a paper-lined plate and place in a warm oven. Repeat until all the mixture is used.
4. Chop the cucumber finely and add to the tzatziki.
5. Place fritters on serving plates. Top with rocket leaves, tzatziki and smoked salmon slices.
   Serves 4

Minestrone soup

2 tbsp olive oil

3 slices pancetta, chopped

2 brown onions, chopped

1 leek sliced

1 carrot chopped

2 sticks celery chopped

2 cloves garlic, chopped

2 zucchinis diced

400 g can crushed tomatoes

1.5 L chicken stock

2 cups water

2 cups baby spinach leaves

120 g small pasta (orzo)

400 g can canellini beans, rinsed and drained

2 tbsp chopped flat-leaf parsley or basil

fresh ground pepper

fresh shaved parmesan to serve

1. Heat oil in a large saucepan over low heat. Add the pancetta and cook, stirring, for 2 minutes. Add the onion, leek, carrot, celery and garlic. Cook, stirring, for 7 to 8 minutes, or until softened.
2. Add the zucchini and tomatoes and stir for 2 minutes. Add the chicken stock and water. Bring to the boil, skim off any scum, reduce the heat and simmer for 30 minutes.
3. Add spinach and pasta and simmer for 20 minutes, stirring occasionally.

4. Add the beans and parsley and extra water or stock if necessary, but not too much because this is a thick soup. Season with pepper and cook for a further 10 minutes.

5. Ladle the soup into bowls and sprinkle with parmesan.

   Serves 6

Chicken avocado bocconcini rolls

2 mini bake-at-home rolls (preferably wholegrain)

20 g avocado

40 g cooked chicken (skinless)

20 g bocconcini sliced

1 Roma tomato, quartered

1. Heat rolls as per packet instructions.

2. Spread avocado on both sides of each roll, and then arrange chicken, boconcini and tomato on each roll.

3. Serve immediately.

Serves 1

Smoked salmon and capers on rye

40 g French bread stick

20 g light philly cheese

60 g smoked salmon

3 tsp capers

1. Slice the French stick into three pieces and spread philly evenly over all three slices.

2. Arrange smoked salmon and capers on top and serve immediately.

Serves 1

Haloumi pizza

20 g reduced-fat haloumi cheese
1 tbsp light hummus (see recipe)
1 small single serve pizza base (50 g)
1 tbsp tomato paste
shake of Italian herbs
4 semi-dried tomatoes
1 mushroom, sliced

1. Cut the haloumi cheese into strips, lightly brown in a hot pan and set aside.
2. Spread hummus over the pizza base and top with tomato paste and herbs. Arrange sun-dried tomatoes and mushrooms over hummus, then place strips of cooked haloumi on top.
3. Bake in a hot oven for 5 to 10 minutes, until the base turns a golden colour.
4. Serve with a side salad.
   Serves 1

Greek lamb salad

300 g lamb
160 g dry bow tie pasta
200 g zucchini, thinly sliced lengthwise
2 cups lettuce

Marinade

1 tsp olive oil
1 tsp garlic
1 tsp rosemary
1½ tbsp lemon juice

Yoghurt dressing

100 g low-fat natural yoghurt
1 tbsp lemon juice
1 tsp chopped garlic

1. For Marinade, place all the ingredients in a glass jar and shake, mixing well.
2. For Yoghurt dressing, just before serving mix all the ingredients together well.
3. Place lamb in a glass dish and pour over the marinade. Put in the fridge and allow to stand at least 2 hours.
4. Cook pasta as per directions on the packet. Set aside.
5. Place marinated lamb on a hot plate of barbecue and cook as desired. Remove from heat and let the lamb sit for 2 minutes. Thinly slice the lamb.
6. Place zucchini on a hot plate and cook on both sides.
7. Arrange lettuce, pasta, zucchini and lamb on a plate and drizzle with yoghurt dressing.
   Serves 4

121

Green beans with chilli

2 tbsp olive oil
2 large leeks, sliced
3–4 cloves garlic, chopped
4–6 Roma tomatoes, roughly chopped
2–3 (or to taste) red chillies, chopped
500 g green beans, topped and tailed

1. Heat olive oil over moderate heat in a large casserole. Add leeks and garlic and cook gently until they are softened.
2. Mix through the chopped tomatoes and chillies and cook gently for 2 to 3 minutes.
3. Add the beans and stir through the mixture.
4. Turn the heat to low, put a lid on the casserole and cook, stirring occasionally for 15 to 20 minutes, until the beans are tender but retain their colour and a bit of crunch. Serve immediately or cold as a salad or side dish.
   Serves 4–6

Salad niçoise

1 red onion, cut into thin wedges
250 g cherry tomatoes, halved
olive oil spray
freshly ground black pepper, to taste
400 g baby potatoes, halved
250 g green beans, topped and tailed
4 fresh tuna steaks, about 100 g each or 400 g can good-quality tuna
100 g rocket leaves

Dressing
2 tbsp fresh squeezed lemon juice
1 tbsp wholegrain or Dijon mustard
2 tsp olive oil
pinch of sugar
salt and pepper, to taste

1. For Dressing: whisk all the ingredients together and season with salt and pepper.
2. Preheat oven to 200°C.
3. Put onion and tomatoes on a baking tray and spray with olive oil. Season with freshly ground pepper and toss to coat. Roast for 10 to 15 minutes until tender.
4. Steam potatoes for about 10 minutes. Add the beans and steam for about 2 minutes, until the potatoes are tender but holding their shape and the beans are bright green and tender. Remove from the steamer and drain.

5. Heat a grill pan or a heavy-based frying pan and spray with olive oil. Add the tuna and sear both sides, about 30 seconds. You can cook it through but it will taste and look better if you just sear it.

6. Gently toss the rocket in with the beans, potatoes, tomatoes and onions in a large bowl or on a platter and drizzle with the dressing. Arrange the fish on top and put in the middle of the table for people to help themselves.

Serves 4

Healthy caesar salad

60 g crusty bread roll, sliced
olive oil
75 g smoked skinless chicken
1 large egg, hard boiled
1 baby cos lettuce (160 g), washed
1–2 anchovies, drained and chopped, for serving

Dressing
1 egg yolk
1 tsp oil
2 tsp Dijon mustard
2 tsp lemon juice
1 tsp garlic
pinch salt and pepper

1. For Dressing: mix all ingredients together well with a hand-held blender or food processor.
2. Lightly spray the bread roll with oil and bake in a hot oven for 3 to 5 minutes until golden.
3. Break up smoked chicken into small pieces, slice eggs into quarters, and arrange with lettuce into two bowls. Add anchovies on top.
4. Pour dressing evenly over each salad and serve immediately.
   Serves 2

125

Roasted vegetable, cannellini bean and feta salad

300 g pumpkin

200 g eggplant

10 cherry tomatoes

1 tsp oil

1 tbsp honey

410 g can cannellini beans (washed)

4 cups mixed green leaves

150 g low-fat feta (cubed)

1 cup rocket leaves

Dressing

¼ cup white vinegar

¼ cup caster sugar

1 tbsp soy sauce

2 tsp sesame oil

1. For Dressing: combine all the ingredients in a saucepan and stir over low heat until sugar is dissolved. Cool and set aside.
2. Cut pumpkin and eggplant into chunks, and slice cherry tomatoes in half.
3. Mix oil and honey together and heat for few seconds in a microwave until thin.
4. Arrange pumpkin, eggplant and tomatoes on a tray and brush with honey and oil. Roast in a hot oven (200°C) for 30 to 40 minutes, until cooked through and golden (remove tomatoes if they start to blacken).
5. Place beans, greens, roasted vegetables and feta in bowl and toss. Pour over dressing and serve immediately.

Serves 4

Prawn and avocado salad

1 cup lettuce, washed
30 g avocado, chopped
100 g mango, sliced
100 g shelled prawns (leave tails on)

Seafood sauce

1 tbsp light mayonnaise
½ tbsp tomato sauce

1. For Seafood sauce: mix the mayonnaise and tomato sauce together well.
2. Arrange lettuce in a bowl and add avocado and mango and toss.
3. Barbecue prawns on a flat grill lightly sprayed with olive oil.
4. Arrange prawns in the salad bowl with tails up and drizzle with seafood sauce.

   Serves 1

Zucchini quiche

1 onion, finely chopped
125 g rindless eye bacon
2 large zucchinis (approx. 300 g), grated
1 medium carrot, grated
70 g low-fat cheese, grated
1½ cup self-raising flour
1 tbp olive oil
5 eggs, lightly beaten
salt and pepper, to taste

1. Microwave or lightly fry onion and bacon for one minute.
2. Combine onion and bacon with zucchini, carrot and cheese.
3. Sift flour, add oil and eggs and season with salt and pepper and mix well. Add in onion mixture.
4. Pour into well-greased muffin trays and bake at 180°C for 40 minutes.
   Makes 12 quiches; serves 6

Chickpea and sweet potato frittata

150 g sweet potato, thinly sliced

1 onion, finely chopped

olive oil, for frying

2 Roma tomatoes, chopped

1 cup mixed frozen peas and corn

100 g can chickpeas, washed

6 eggs

2 tbp reduced-fat milk

30 g parmesan cheese, shaved

1. In a non-stick frying pan, sautee sweet potato with onion in a small amount of olive oil until potato is softened.

2. Add tomatoes, peas, corn and chickpeas, and stir-fry for 2 minutes.

3. Beat eggs and milk together. Poor over vegetables and simmer slowly on a low heat until almost set. Arrange parmesan cheese on top and lightly brown under the grill.

4. Serve with a small side salad.

Serves 4

Bean salad

400 g can cannelloni beans
400 g can chick peas
400 g can butter beans
1 red onion, finely chopped
1 small Lebanese cucumber, finely chopped
1 red or yellow capsicum, finely chopped
1 bunch coriander (or parsley), finely chopped
juice of 2 or 3 lemons

1. Drain and rinse the beans and put into a bowl. Add red onion, capsicum, cucumber and coriander. Mix gently.
2. Pour just enough of the lemon juice over the salad to moisten but not overwhelm the taste.

   Serves 6 to 8

Not only is this recipe yummy, it's virtually fat free.

Mango Salsa

1 small red onion, finely chopped
1 red or yellow capsicum, finely chopped
1 small Lebanese cucumber, finely chopped
2 large mangoes, roughly chopped
1 bunch fresh coriander (or parsley), finely chopped
400 g can chickpeas
juice of 2 or 3 lemons, or to taste

1. Put red onion, capsicum and cucumber in a bowl and add mangoes and coriander.
2. Drain and rinse chickpeas. Mix in gently with other ingredients.
3. Pour over enough lemon juice to moisten but not overwhelm the flavours, and serve.

Serves 6–8

Dinner

This is an excellent time to sit with family to chat and savour the main meal of the day. A rule of thumb for serving portions of food on your dinner plates is one-quarter should hold the protein (seafood, chicken, other meats or legumes), and one-quarter is set aside for the slow-release starch foods (rice, pasta, new potatoes – a healthy serving is between half to one cup for the main meal). The other half of the plate contains . . . yes, you've guessed it . . . fresh vegetables and salad items.

Vegetable tomato sauce

500 g ripe tomatoes, chopped
1 small butternut pumpkin, peeled and chopped
1 carrot, chopped
1 zucchini, chopped
2 cups chicken stock
1 clove garlic
½ onion, finely chopped
400 g can tomatoes

This is a good basic sauce for pizzas and pastas and bakes and it can be stored in containers and frozen.

1. Place tomatoes, pumpkin, carrot and zucchini on a tray lined with baking paper. Roast in a moderate oven for 30 minutes.
2. Place baked vegetables in a food processor and process with 1 cup of stock.
3. Strain liquid through a sieve and place liquid in a saucepan and add garlic, onion, tomatoes and remaining stock. Simmer gently for 30 minutes.

Hummus

440 g can chickpeas drained
2 tbsp lemon juice
2 tbsp tahini
½ tsp cumin
2 tsp olive oil
1 clove garlic, crushed

1. Place all ingredients in a food processor and blend until the mix reaches the required consistency. This recipe makes approximately 2 cups. Each serve is 4 tablespoons.

San choy bow wraps

2 tbsp extra virgin olive oil

1 onion, finely diced

2 cloves garlic, crushed

1 tsp grated fresh ginger

500 g skinless chicken, minced

2 tsp cornflour

½ cup chicken stock

½ cup chopped water chestnuts

2 tbsp soy sauce

iceberg or cos lettuce cups

bean sprouts, to serve

1. Heat oil in a frying pan or wok, stir-fry onion, garlic and ginger for 2 minutes. Add chicken mince and stir-fry until golden.
2. Mix cornflour into stock and add to pan. Add chestnuts and soy sauce and simmer for a few minutes, until thickened.
3. Serve on lettuce cups and top with fresh bean sprouts.
   Serves 4

Spicy lentil patty stacks

4 slices eggplant

4 large field mushrooms

olive oil spray

1 cup brown lentils, washed and drained

3 cups water

1 tsp curry powder

1 tsp cumin powder

1 tsp coriander powder

1 tsp oil

1 carrot, peeled and finely chopped

2 tsp crushed garlic

1 onion, finely chopped

1½ cup bread crumbs

2 tbsp plain flour

2 tbsp tomato paste

1 tbsp soy sauce

4 cups greens, wilted

1. Place eggplant and mushroom on a baking tray and spray lightly with olive oil. Bake in moderate oven until just cooked through, about 20 minutes.
2. Place lentils in a saucepan with water, curry powder and spices. Bring to a boil and simmer for about 30 minutes, until lentils are just soft. Set aside.
3. In a pan add oil, carrot, garlic and onion and and stir-fry until onions are golden. Pour off any remaining liquid from lentils and mash.
4. Add mashed lentils to carrot mixture. Add bread crumbs, flour, tomato paste and soy sauce, and mix well.

5. Roll into six balls and flatten into patties. Place on a tray lined with baking paper and bake at 180°C for 30 to 40 minutes, turning patties halfway through cooking time.

6. Serve with oven-roasted eggplant, field mushrooms and wilted greens.

Makes 4 patties; serves 4

Teriyaki tofu and zucchini

85 g dry thin noodles
olive oil spray
400 g solid tofu, cubed
100 g mushrooms, cut in half
1 cup vegetable stock
4 tbsp teriyaki sauce
1 tsp soy sauce
1 tbsp honey
180 g broccoli florets
80 g green beans, topped, tailed and halved
1 small zucchini, thinly sliced

1. Cook noodles as directed on packet and set aside.
2. Spray a pan with oil and stir-fry tofu until just golden. Add mushrooms, stock, sauces and honey, reduce heat to medium, stirring well until sauce reduces by about a third and thickens. Add broccoli, beans, zucchini and noodles. Mix well and serve immediately.

Serves 4

Chilli salmon steaks with Asian greens

100 ml plain low-fat yoghurt
2 tbsp lemon juice
fresh coriander, chopped, to taste
1 red chilli, chopped
1 tbsp olive oil
600 g fresh Atlantic salmon, cut into four pieces
green salad of baby mesculin, rocket, baby spinach and bean sprouts

1. Mix the yoghurt, lemon juice and coriander in a bowl and set aside.
2. Mix chilli and oil together and lightly rub one side of the salmon steaks with the mix. Lightly brush the cooking surface with oil and barbecue or pan-fry salmon until cooked through, 2–4 minutes each side. If you're a sushi fan, cook for 2 minutes, but if you don't like it raw in the centre, cook for 4 minutes.
3. Mix greens together and drizzle with yoghurt dressing.
4. Serve salmon immediately with salad.
   Serves 4

Green fish curry

1 onion, quartered and separated

½ large sweet potato (150 g), chopped

2 tbsp green curry paste

½ cup chicken stock

1 cup snow peas, sliced in half

300 g thick white fish (mahi mahi or swordfish), cut into small chunks

1 cup reduced-fat milk

2 tsp coconut essence

lime juice, to taste

fish sauce, to taste

1½ cups cooked rice

1. Stir-fry onion and sweet potato in the green curry paste for one minute. Add stock and simmer until sweet potato is soft. Add snow peas and fish and stir-fry for two minutes. Add milk, coconut essence, lime juice and fish sauce.
2. If the sauce is too runny, thicken with cornflour mixed into a small amount of water. Cook for 2–3 minutes until sauce is thickened.
3. Serve with rice.

   Serves 3

Tandoori lamb cutlets with coriander yoghurt dressing

2 tsp low-fat plain yoghurt
1 tbsp Tandoori paste
400 g (approx. 12) lean lamb chops, fat removed
salad or vegetables of your choice

Yoghurt dressing

2 tsp low-fat plain yoghurt
1 tbsp fresh coriander (or coriander paste)
1 tbsp lemon juice

1. For Yoghurt dressing: mix yoghurt, coriander and lemon juice together.
2. Mix plain yoghurt and Tandoori paste together and pour over chops. Refrigerate for 1 hour.
3. Barbecue or grill marinated lamb until tender. Drizzle with yoghurt dressing and serve with a large salad.

   Serves 4

Italian spaghetti and meatballs

500 g beef, minced
1 onion, finely diced
2 cloves garlic, crushed
¼ cup dried breadcrumbs
1 tsp mixed Italian herbs (dried)
1 tsp salt
pinch pepper
1 egg, beaten
500 g spaghetti, cooked

Tomato sauce
olive oil spray
1 onion, finely chopped
400 g can crushed tomatoes
2 tbsp tomato paste
fresh or dried Italian herbs, to taste
salt and pepper, to taste

1. For Tomato sauce: spray the pan with oil and brown onion on medium heat. Add tomatoes and bring to a boil. Add remaining ingredients and simmer until reduced and thickened.
2. Place the mince, onion, garlic, breadcrumbs, herbs, salt and pepper in a bowl. Add egg and mix well.
3. With floured hands roll into balls that are approximately 2 spoonfuls in size.
4. Spray a non-stick pan with oil and fry meatballs until golden, then set aside.
5. Cook spaghetti as per packet instructions and serve with meatballs topped with tomato sauce.

   Makes 25 balls; serves 5

Eggplant and basil parmigiana

3 small eggplants cut into ½–1 cm slices
olive oil in spray can
1 tbsp olive oil
1 medium brown onion, finely chopped
2–3 cloves crushed garlic
2 cups passatta (tomato sauce)
1 can diced Italian tomatoes
150 g crumbled low-fat ricotta cheese
100 g crumbled low-fat feta cheese
100 g grated parmesan cheese
small bunch basil leaves

1. Preheat oven to 180°C. Preheat a barbecue or chargrill plate or grill on medium–high.
2. Spray eggplant slices liberally on both sides with olive oil. Chargrill in batches for 1 to 2 minutes on each side or until tender.
3. Put olive oil, onions and garlic to a pan. Cook gently, stirring occasionally, until the onion is soft (about 5 minutes). Add tomato passatta and tomatoes and simmer gently, about 10 minutes.
4. Layer half the eggplant in the base of an ovenproof dish with the slices overlapping. Sprinkle with half the ricotta, feta, parmesan and basil leaves. Spoon over half the tomato sauce. Top with the remaining grilled eggplant. Scatter the remaining feta and ricotta over the top layer of eggplant, spoon over the remaining tomato sauce and sprinkle with remaining parmesan. Decorate the top with the remaining basil leaves.

5. Bake in the over for 25 to 30 minutes until hot and bubbling. Serve hot or at room temperature.

Serves 4–6

Tuna pasta

500 g dried pasta
1 tbsp olive oil
1 brown onion, chopped
2–4 cloves garlic, finely chopped
400 g can butter beans, drained and rinsed
400 g can cannellini beans, drained and rinsed
1 large can tuna in spring water, drained
1 small jar sliced black Spanish olives, drained
1 small jar capers, drained

1. Cook the pasta in boiling salted water until al dente.
2. In a large, deep frying pan heat olive oil and cook the onions and garlic gently until softened.
3. Combine the beans, tuna, olives and capers with the onion and garlic in the pan. Add a little olive oil to moisten. Gently heat through.
4. Drain the cooked pasta and stir through the bean mixture. Add a bit more olive oil to coat the pasta, if necessary.
5. Serve immediately with a green salad.
   Serves 4–6

Vegetable stacks

1 kg butternut pumpkin, cut in ½-cm slices
1 red and 1 yellow capsicum, cut into strips
olive oil, to drizzle
1 tbsp olive oil
2 green onions
300 g frozen (or fresh) peas
1 can of butter or cannellini beans
150 g rocket
packet of flour tortillas
goats or feta cheese (optional)

Dressing
1 bunch flat-leaf parsley
1–2 tbsp salted capers, rinsed
⅓ cup extra virgin olive oil
1–2 tbsp fresh lemon juice

1. For Dressing: put all the ingredients in a food processor and finely chop.
2. Place pumpkin and capsicum on a baking tray, drizzle with a little olive oil and roast in a hot oven until browned and tender (about 30 minutes).
3. Heat 1 tablespoon olive oil in a pan and gently cook the green onion until soft. Add peas, beans and rocket, and stir until the rocket is wilted.
4. Place pea mixture on a plate, top with half a tortilla, then a layer of pumpkin, another half tortilla, and slices of capsicum. Spoon over the dressing. Sprinkle with goat's cheese if desired.

Serves 4–6

Roast chicken with preserved lemon

1 bunch parsley

1 bunch thyme (or sage) leaves

4 cloves garlic

3–4 wedges of preserved lemon

2–3 tbsp olive oil

1 large organic or free range chicken

1. Preheat oven to 200°C.

2. In a food processor, mix together the parsley, thyme, garlic, preserved lemons and just enough olive oil to make a coarse paste.

3. Put the chicken into a roasting pan and, with your fingers, gently separate the skin from the flesh of the chicken by running your fingers under the skin to loosen it from the flesh. Try not to break the skin. Push the herb mixture into the space between the skin and the flesh. Make sure the mixture gets pushed right down into the legs and is evenly distributed under the skin.

4. Bake in the oven for about an hour or until the juices from the thigh run clear when poked with a fork.

Serves 6

147

Oriental beef stir-fry

500 g premium beef, cut into strips
2 tbsp plain flour
1 onion, quartered and separated
1 tsp sesame or peanut oil
227 g can whole water chestnuts
225 g can bamboo shoots
150 g oriental mushrooms
2 tsp crushed garlic
1 tsp grated ginger
2 tbsp oyster sauce
2 tbsp soy sauce
200 g Hokkien noodles
1 cup beef stock
salad, to serve

1. Place beef and flour in a plastic bag and shake.
2. Cook the onion and beef in peanut oil until just browned, then remove from pan.
3. Add chestnuts, bamboo shoots and mushrooms and stir-fry for 1 minute. Add garlic, ginger and sauces, stirring on low heat.
4. Return meat to pan with noodles and beef stock, stirring until liquid reduces and thickens.
5. Serve with salad.

   Serves 4

Spaghetti marinara

200 g Atlantic salmon steak

250 g (approx. 12) shelled prawns

100 g calamari hood, cut into rings

2 tsp olive oil

1 onion, chopped

2 tsp crushed garlic

1 cup white wine

400 g can crushed tomatoes

dried Italian herbs, to taste

1 tsp parsley

2 bay leaves

1 tsp sugar

1 tbsp tomato paste

170 g dry spaghetti

1. In a non-stick frying pan, satuee batches of seafood in oil for 1 minute, remove from pan and set aside.

2. Add onions and garlic to the pan and fry for 1 minute. Add white wine, tomatoes and herbs and simmer for 5 minutes. Add sugar and tomato paste, stirring well until sugar dissolves, about 1 minute. Remove from heat.

3. Cook spaghetti as per packet directions.

4. Return seafood to tomato sauce mixture and warm through.

5. Serve over spaghetti.

Serves 4

149

Pesto-crusted whiting

2 tbsp dry breadcrumbs
1 tbsp pesto
600 g (approx. 8) whiting fillets

Pesto

20 g pine nuts, lightly roasted
1 bunch fresh basil leaves, washed and torn
10 g parmesan cheese, grated
2 tbsp olive oil
1 tsp garlic

1. For Pesto: place all ingredients in a food processor and blend until smooth. Makes 130 g (approx ½ cup) of paste. Extra pesto can be stored in the refrigerator or frozen.
2. Mix breadcrumbs and pesto in a bowl.
3. Cover whiting in pesto and barbecue on a hot plate until cooked, about 1 minute each side.
   Serves 2

Chicken and asparagus risotto

1½ tbsp oil
400 g chicken fillets, sliced
2 cups mushrooms, thickly sliced
1 onion, finely sliced
2 cups arborio rice
½ cup dry white wine
4–5 cups vegetable or chicken stock
1 bunch asparagus, chopped
⅓ cup grated parmesan cheese
3 tbsp freshly squeezed lemon juice

1. Heat oil in a pan on high heat and fry chicken and mushrooms until lightly golden. Remove from the pan and set aside.
2. Add onion to pan and fry for 2 to 3 minutes. Add rice and cook for 2 minutes, stirring continuously. Add wine and continue stirring until absorbed.
3. Add stock, one cup at a time, until all is absorbed, stirring regularly. This step is crucial for a lovely, light and fluffy risotto, so be careful not to add stock too quickly. Each cup can take a few minutes to absorb. When rice has a creamy consistency add chicken, mushrooms and asparagus.
4. Stir in parmesan and lemon juice and garnish with a few thin slices of parmesan on top before serving.

Serves 7

Pumpkin and feta risotto

300 g pumpkin, peeled and cubed
olive oil spray
1½ tbsp oil
1 onion, finely sliced
2 cups arborio rice
½ cup dry white wine
4–5 cups vegetable stock
1 bunch asparagus, chopped
2 cups mushrooms, thickly sliced
⅓ cup grated parmesan cheese
100 g reduced-fat feta cheese

1. Arrange pumpkin on a baking tray, spray lightly with oil and bake until golden.
2. Heat oil in a pan and fry onion for 2 to 3 minutes. Add rice and cook for 2 minutes, stirring continuously. Add wine and continue stirring until absorbed.
3. Add vegetable stock, one cup at a time, until all is absorbed, stirring regularly. When rice has a creamy consistency add pumpkin, asparagus and mushrooms.
4. Stir in parmesan and feta and garnish with a few thin slices of parmesan on top before serving.

   Serves 4

Napoli Pizza

1 family size pizza base
4 tbsp basic tomato sauce
2 tbsp cream cheese
½ medium avocado
100 g ham or pastrami
salsa
½ cup grated tasty or mozzarella cheese
baby spinach leaves

1. Arrange ingredients over pizza base and finish with a sprinkle of tasty cheese. Cook in a medium oven and grill until cheese is golden. The beauty of this pizza is that it can be used as a light lunch or served as the main meal.
Serves 4

Seafood pizza

1 family size pizza base
4 tbsp tomato paste
100 g feta cheese
baby corn spears
2 cups fresh seafood marinara mix
1 avocado, sliced
cherry tomatoes, sliced in half

1. Cover base with tomato paste. Arrange all the ingredients over. Cook in a moderately hot oven for 15 to 20 minutes, until golden.
Serves 4

153

Asian drumsticks

1 tbsp hoi sin sauce

1 tbsp soy

1 tbsp honey

1 tsp peanut oil

1 tsp garlic

400g (approx. 8) small 'lovely legs' skinless chicken drumsticks

2 cups cooked rice, to serve

salad or vegetables, to serve

1. Combine hoi sin, soy, honey, oil and garlic in a small bowl and set aside.
2. Place chicken drumsticks in a single layer on baking paper and brush with sauce mixture, coating both sides. Place in a 200°C oven and roast for 35 to 40 minutes or until chicken juices are clear when flesh is pierced with a knife.
3. Serve on rice with salad or vegetables.
   Serves 4

Chicken, baby corn and bok choy stir-fry

1 onion, diced
1 tsp grated ginger
1 tsp garlic
1 tsp sesame oil
400 g chicken breast, sliced
4 bunches baby bok choy
1 cup sweet corn spears
1 tbsp soy sauce
1 cup chicken stock
1 tbsp cornflour, optional
1 tsp black pepper
2 cups cooked rice, to serve

1. In pan cook onion, ginger and garlic in sesame oil until fragrant. Add chicken and stir-fry for 2 minutes, until golden. Remove from pan and set aside.
2. Add bok choy and sweet corn to pan and stir-fry until leaves have wilted.
3. Return chicken to pan and add soy sauce and chicken stock and simmer for 1 minute. If you desire a thicker consistency, mix 1 tablespoon of cornflour in cold water in a cup and slowly add to pan and mix through. Season with black pepper to taste.
4. Serve with rice.
   Serves 4

Sea perch with lime and chilli marinade

150 g sea perch fillets
1 large cob corn, cut into 4 slices
rocket leaves, washed
lime wedges

Marinade

1 tsp grated or minced ginger
1 tsp olive oil
1 tsp fresh or concentrate lime juice
1 tbsp sweet chilli sauce

1. For Marinade: place all ingredients in a jar and shake well.
2. Pour marinade over fillets and set aside in refrigerator for at least 1 hour.
3. Barbecue fillets on a grilling plate until cooked through, 1–2 minutes each side. Remove from heat and let sit for 2 minutes.
4. Add corn cobs to barbecue and cook to taste.
5. Slice perch into thick slices and arrange on rocket and serve with cob of corn and lime wedges.

Serves 1

Part 4
Calmer

Chapter 10

Benefits of being calm

When you face a challenge or threat, how do you respond? Be honest. Are you likely to objectively view the situation and then act accordingly, or fly off the handle, lashing out at all and sundry. These two quite different responses are among a whole range of feelings and reactions you may have when events, real or perceived, provoke you. Stress does that to people. While challenging situations beyond your control and uncontrolled responses by you to those situations can contribute to long-term health problems, it is important to understand that you need some stress to perform optimally. Not all stress is bad.

What is stress?

Put simply, stress causes you to experience changes in your hormone levels and the effects of this include an increase in your heart rate and blood pressure. Badly managed stress may be associated with a variety of symptoms such as poor concentration, sweaty palms, muscular tension, and an inability to function properly. Diabetes, heart disease, hypertension, cancer, gastrointestinal and immune system problems are all aggravated when stress goes unchecked. But the stress response allows you to respond to threats or challenges – you fight the threat or flee from it.

Fight or flight is very effective if you occasionally face the threat of a hungry tiger or a spear-wielding savage, or even an on-coming car swerving out of control. You deal with the problem and either survive or don't. The important thing here is you deal with it or avoid the thing that is stressing you. But many of the threats and challenges that create stress in our lives today, like traffic jams or an unsympathetic boss, may be ongoing, which creates a situation that is essentially inappropriate and unhealthy. In the modern working environment the thing that causes stress may be difficult to avoid or deal with and that is what creates an ongoing stress response in you.

Calming ways for a better life

If you don't deal with this stress effectively, not only will the ongoing stress response affect your health, you are more liable to engage in negative behaviours such as drinking too much, smoking and comfort eating, which also affect your health and wellbeing and tend to make you feel like you have no control over your life, your stress levels and/or your behaviour. This in turn can lead to anxiety and depression as well as weight gain.

Learning about yourself, and how you deal with stress is vitally important to making your life calmer, and preventing the negative aspects of stress. Teaching yourself to relax and calm down is a skill and, like any other skill, takes practice. So take the time to do that. There are a number of benefits to being calm:

- It improves the functioning of your immune system. Numerous studies have shown that stress immediately increases the output of hormones that have a negative effect on your white blood cells, which you need to work well for a good immune response. The nice part here, though, is that when the thing that stresses you is removed, this situation is quite rapidly addressed by your body and everything returns to normal. So when you get stressed, if you act to reduce the stress it will have a positive and rapid effect.

- It slows your heart rate. A chronically elevated heart rate means your heart has to work too hard and this can lead to heart disease.

- It lowers blood pressure. High heart rates cause elevations in blood pressure which also means that your heart has to work too hard and this can lead to chronic high blood pressure and heart disease. Stress hormones have a direct effect on blood pressure so learning to deal with stress will reduce the hormone response and, hence, the downstream effects of those hormones.

- It slows your breathing rate. When you breathe rapidly, your breath tends to be shallow. Slow, deep breathing stimulates a relaxation response.

- It increases blood flow to major muscles. When this happens muscles release tension and function better.

- It reduces pain responses. Tense muscles can lead to chronic pain as the tension feeds back to the brain and causes psychological tension which, in turn feeds back to increase muscle tension. Relaxation breaks the cycle.

- It improves concentration. It is difficult to concentrate on a task when you are over-aroused (stressed). Relaxation allows you to pay attention to the important things in life – not the things that make you stressed.

- It reduces anger and frustration. These negative emotions focus your attention inappropriately and make it difficult for you to focus on solving problems. They may also increase your risk of heart disease. When you relax and approach the issues calmly, you are reducing your stress response and enhancing your ability to deal with the source of the anger and frustration

163

and/or simply make it less important and therefore less able to stimulate a negative response in you.

- It boosts confidence in your ability to handle problems. When you learn to manage your stress levels and be calm, it helps you when you are addressing problems but it also aids in developing your confidence in your ability to solve problems. After all, you've learned to manage your stress, so you can pretty much learn to manage most things!

TAKE-HOME MESSAGE

Too much uncontrolled stress can negatively affect your physical and psychological health, sleep and body composition. Learning how to control stress and your responses to stressors has positive effects on all aspects of your life. There is a wide variety of techniques to use that help to reduce the stress response and one of these techniques will work for you.

Chapter 11

Ten tips for a calmer you

There are many ways to induce a state of relaxation. One of them is bound to work for you. But, you also have to put in the effort. Learning how to reduce stress is a skill that you learn to master with practice. So persist and you will find it becomes easier and easier.

The first step is to recognise when your stress levels are too high. Learn to monitor muscle tension, especially in the muscles of the shoulders and neck. Does your heart race or pound in your chest? Are you breathing rapidly and shallowly? Are you short-tempered and impatient? The signs will vary from individual to individual so the first thing you should do is learn to check yourself: your mood and how your body feels.

You will learn to pick up the signs when stress is getting to you and then you can follow some of these strategies to manage it. The added benefit of these activities is that they are not only effective at reducing stress, they also help to make you a healthier, happier person.

1. Exercise

Many studies have shown that regular exercise reduces anxiety and depression and improves thinking. The reason for this is not clear but the fact that we don't really understand the why, does not reduce the benefits of the how. Certainly part of the answer is improved blood flow and overall cardiovascular function.

Exercise has a number of useful benefits in terms of dealing with stress:

- it enhances your mood and reduces anxiety
- you have a better sense of control over yourself and your environment
- you feel good about yourself
- it distracts you from the problems causing the stress
- it reduces (after exercise) heart rate and blood pressure
- it gives you time out from your daily hassles – me time!
- it provides you with social interaction
- it provides you with the physical capacity to face problems
- it makes you healthier and a healthy person is a happy person.

The best thing about it is that it doesn't appear to matter (from the psychological point of view) what sort of exercise you do. So, if you do *LifeSprints*, great. But strength training, Pilates, yoga, swimming, going for a walk – whatever – will also do the trick.

2. Avoid caffeine, nicotine and sugar

These stimulants act in the same way as other things that create stress. They increase your heart rate and blood pressure and can cause changes in your body's stress hormone levels. The recommended dose of caffeine for non-pregnant adults is less than 600 mg/day, which is equivalent to two strong cups of coffee. So, if you enjoy a morning latte, don't feel you have to give it up. But do remember that chocolate, tea, cola-type soft drinks, etc., contain caffeine and you may be getting more caffeine than you realise.

Cigarettes (nicotine) are bad for you on all levels and cigarette smoke is a major environmental stressor. If you do smoke, try to cut down and get some help to give it up entirely. New scientific data indicates that cigarette smoke not only causes heart disease, high blood pressure, strokes and a whole range of cancers but it is implicated in the development of liver disease.

And if you need a sugar hit, get it from fresh fruit. Fruit contains sugars as well as many nutrients that are good for you. So bite into an apple today, and leave the chocolate for occasional, special treats.

3. Change the situation

If you are in a situation that is untenable and you can't change the factors causing your stress, find ways to remove yourself from the situation. For example, if your boss is a bully, get yourself moved to another department under a different boss or find other employment. If you do change jobs, make sure you have a new job to go to before you resign from the present one, otherwise you simply change one stressor (the bully) for another (unemployment).

4. Change your attitude to the stressor

This can be a challenge but, if you meet it, it can be very rewarding. If you change your response towards the thing that creates your stress it no longer has that effect on you. An example of this is being stuck in peak-hour traffic and someone cuts in front of you and swears at you. You have a choice: you can respond with rude gestures and swear and try to cut them off, or you can just ignore them, smile and wave and make room for them to get into the lane in front of you.

A helpful strategy here is to try to imagine the possible events that lead to that person behaving in that way. For example, they have had a bad day at the office and their supervisor has given them a warning and they don't feel that their supervisor is being fair so they take it out on the others – in this case other road users. If your response is sympathetic, you are less likely to get distressed by their behaviour.

5. Manage your time more effectively

Poor time management is a huge stress factor. If you are always scrambling to meet deadlines, you put yourself in the position of playing catch-up all the time. If you are a procrastinator, try to find out why you avoid certain tasks and then find strategies to change those behaviours. Get some help. Reward yourself when you do something on time as an encouragement.

Time management is a skill and it can be learned. There is a wealth of information out there (especially online) about it. The address for the University of New South Wales' time management website is http://www.lc.unsw.edu.au/onlib/time.html and there are links to other websites that will help you to develop strategies to improve your time-management skills.

6. Give yourself time out

We all need 'me' time. What that will entail will vary from person to person. It may be going for a walk, having a bubble bath, listening to music, going to a movie, reading a book, having a manicure, doing pottery, going surfing, enjoying coffee with friends – the list is endless. Every week schedule at least one period where you do something you enjoy just for the sake of that enjoyment. And don't feel guilty about it!

Avoid using food, especially comfort food like chocolate, as your me time reward. This is likely to lead to you feeling like you have transgressed and reinforces the notion that food is comforting and rewarding. Food is essential to life but if you use it as a reward, you can reinforce negative eating behaviours.

7. Practise mental imagery, meditation, breathing

Just taking a deep breath will slow your heart rate, and lowering your heart rate will automatically reduce your blood pressure, all of which will act as de-stressors. Visualise a tranquil scene and breathe slowly. You can easily find a course to learn how to meditate, or do some yoga classes to learn how to breathe properly. Simple contract/relax exercises, where you systematically tighten then relax the muscles in your body, will also help here.

8. Think positively

We all have negative thought patterns at times. Instead of focusing on the negatives in your life, try to think about the positive aspects. You can change your thought patterns. If you find yourself thinking negatively about something, practise changing that into a positive thought. For example, you are sitting in traffic and not going anywhere. A negative response to this is to get frustrated and angry and curse your fellow road users. A positive response is to put on your favourite CD, or listen to the radio, phone a friend (using hands-free, of course) or (this is my favourite) give yourself a bit of a manicure. That old saying, every cloud has a silver lining, is true and you can find something good in everything if you make the effort.

9. Eat well

Part 3 gave you lots of information about the Med–Asian diet. It contains lots of fresh, whole food, which provides the building blocks for a healthy body and, in particular, a healthy immune system. This great tasting food is packed with lots of antioxidants to counteract the effects of environmental stressors. Being healthy in and of itself reduces stress because illness and injury act as stressors.

Eating well is not just a function of eating good food. It should also have a social function wherein you share your food with friends and family. Social interaction is extremely important for your wellbeing. The opportunity to discuss, over a nice meal, the day's events, is a de-stressor in itself. So enjoy good, well-prepared food and the people you share it with.

10. Sleep well

Sleeping well is important. Treat your bed as your sanctuary. It is not a workplace or a TV viewing station. It is a place to sleep and to enjoy your partner. Poor sleep acts like a stressor and can stimulate the stress response if not addressed.

Studies have shown that those who have too much or too little sleep are more prone to obesity, and poor quality sleep can make the rest of your life a misery. You need to work out the right amount of sleep you need. Seven to eight hours appears to be the optimal amount of sleep, but monitor your sleeping habits over a week and then add up the hours and divide by seven. This will give you the average amount of sleep you need each night. If you are getting more or less than that, you should adjust your sleeping times.

If you have poor sleep patterns here are a number of strategies to help:

- Avoid food and alcohol for at least an hour before sleep. Going to bed too full or hungry will make it difficult to fall asleep and will disturb your sleep once you get there. Alcohol can dehydrate you and acts like a diuretic, so your sleep is disturbed by the need to have a drink (of water) and/or to go to the toilet.
- Don't smoke before bed – preferably not at all. Nicotine acts as a stimulant and makes it more difficult to fall asleep and stay asleep so it is best avoided close to bed time.
- Exercise either in the morning or in the late afternoon or in the morning. Exercise during the day (before 4 pm) does not appear to directly affect sleep patterns but physically fit people generally have better sleeping behaviours. Exercise between 4 and 6 pm that is vigorous enough to make

you sweat has been shown to improve the quality of your sleep. Bear in mind, exercising late at night appears to disrupt sleep, probably because of the increase in body temperature that accompanies vigorous exercise.

- Have a set time for bed and stick to it. Humans are creatures of habit and if you establish a habit of going to sleep at a particular time, your internal clock will tell you that it is time to go to sleep and you will go to sleep if you give yourself the opportunity. Anyone who has travelled overseas can tell you about how effective your internal clock is. But, we know it can also be adjusted – after all, you don't suffer from jet lag forever. So what you need to do is train your internal clock.

- Sleeping in is a nice luxury on a Sunday morning but keep it as a once-a-week treat. On all the other days get up early enough to get adequate sunlight and to have time to do all the things you want/have to do. Sunlight is important for psychological health and you need it to help in the formation of vitamin D in the body. Morning sun is great because the UV index is low up to 8 am.

- Avoid using your bedroom as an amusement parlour (unless the amusement is sex) as games and other distracters prevent you from relaxing and falling asleep. Your body needs to calm down sufficiently to transition into sleep and games or a TV program may just act as stimulants rather than the opposite. Also, if you fall asleep with the TV on you are not getting a good sleep as the noise will affect the quality of your sleep.

- If you have trouble getting to sleep, try some progressive relaxation activities (see Chapter 12), deep breathing and/or meditation, rather than lying there feeling frustrated. Fidgeting and worrying about falling asleep will simply keep you awake. Relax, and let your body do the rest.

- Get professional help and advice if you need it as worrying about not sleeping compounds the problems.

TAKE-HOME MESSAGE

Techniques to calm yourself, such as controlled breathing, progressive muscle relaxation, guided imagery and exercise, have the ability to reduce stress and anxiety. Combined with exercise and healthy eating, stress-management techniques provide the basis for a healthy lifestyle. Good quality sleep is important to your psychological and physical health and reducing your stress levels will help you to achieve this.

Chapter 12

Relaxation exercises

Why you need to relax has been discussed in the previous chapter. Here we are going to look at how you can do that – and sometimes it's easier said than done. Be prepared to try several strategies and persist until you find what works for you. Learning to control your stress is a skill that takes practice. You will find some activities are more suited to you than others.

Progressive relaxation

If you Google 'Jacobson relaxation' you will get a number of websites that walk you through this process. Essentially the idea is that mental anxiety/stress causes muscular tension, and if you release the muscular tension, you will reduce your anxiety/stress. It works. It is also a useful technique when you are having difficulty falling asleep. In a nutshell:

- get into a comfortable position
- starting with your feet, tense those muscles, and then quickly relax them
- work up your legs, contracting and relaxing the muscles of your calf and thighs, then do the muscles of the trunk, then shoulders, then arms, then neck and face
- to finish off, tense your whole body, then let it flop – lovely!

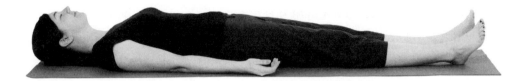

Deep breathing

Most of us breathe shallowly, especially when we are tense. A quick stress relief is to breathe deeply through your nose. Make the breath deep enough to fill your lungs to the very bottom. Hold for a second, and then slowly release the breath through your mouth. Let the tension go with the breath. Repeat a couple of times and feel yourself relax.

Visualisation/imagery

This process involves visualising yourself in a situation that is warm, secure, safe and relaxing. The place will vary from person to person but the following will give you an idea:

- imagine yourself at the top of the stairs
- step down and each time you step down take a deep breath in and out, releasing the tension in your body
- when you get to the bottom of the stairs, imagine a pathway winding through a warm, sunny paddock full of flowers
- walk down the path until you come to a pond full of lily pads

- step into the warm water and lie down on a lily pad (they are as big as your imagination)
- feel the warm sun and a light breeze running over your body
- keep breathing deeply
- feel the warm water and the lily pad supporting you as you float on the surface
- stay there as long as you need to
- when you are ready, get out of the water and walk back through the paddock to the stairs
- as you walk up the stairs, start to expand your awareness to the outside world and, when you are ready, open your eyes and face the world afresh.

Other imagery options are floating on a cloud, walking through a garden, sailing on the ocean, lying on a beach. Any occasion or environment, imaginary or real, in which you feel happy and comfortable and not threatened by anything, will work here.

Meditation

Meditation, in some senses, defies definition. Some texts call it mindfulness and some maintain that it is focusing on a particular object, sound or thought. People use prayer, mantras, musical chants and a variety of other techniques or objects to focus their attention on the present, the here and now. One of the effects of this is to prevent focus on those thoughts or activities that create stress and thus induce a state of relaxation.

Meditation is practised by many different groups from yoga practitioners to religious faiths. Learning to meditate may be guided by finding a suitable teacher. You can, however, teach yourself to meditate with these seven keys.

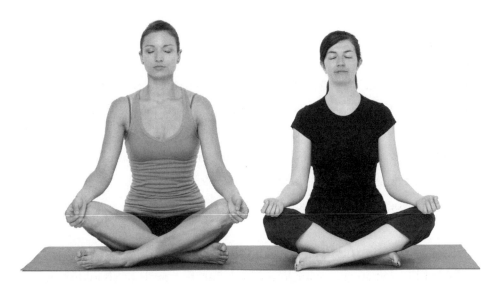

1. Find a special spot for your meditation. It may be in your bedroom or in the garden or on a beach. What is important is that this is your special place and you meditate here.

2. Prepare yourself. Have a shower or wash your face and hands. Put on loose comfortable clothes and take off your shoes.

3. Sit in a comfortable position with your back straight. Take six or seven deep breaths, completely filling your lungs, and then let the air out slowly through your mouth.

4. Take it slowly. Initially five minutes may be enough. Gradually build up the time as you need.

5. Meditate at a suitable time. Practise daily. First thing in the morning prepares you for the day. At the end of the day, it will allow you to unwind and rid yourself of the day's detritus. Avoid meditating when you are hungry or full after a meal as your body's demands will make it difficult.

6. Use gentle music to soften your soul and guide you to relaxation.

7. Breathe deeply. When you breathe in, breathe in peace. When you breathe out, breathe out all your tension.

Yoga

Yoga is an excellent way to learn how to relax, meditate and stretch out tense muscles. Traditionally yoga was developed as a form of meditation and has grown outside India as a gentle way to exercise (Hatha Yoga). If you feel this would be of use to you, the best thing to do is to find a local practitioner and enjoy the classes with other likeminded people.

Try this yoga relaxation technique.

1. Place a matt on the floor with the short edge touching a wall. Set up a folded blanket so that your lower back can rest on it (it shouldn't be too high). You are going to lie down on the matt with your feet up on the wall.
2. To get your hips close to the wall, sit on the blanket and scoot your backside as close to the wall as you can, then swing your legs to rest on the wall. If your hamstrings are tight, focus on getting your feet on the wall rather than the entire leg.
3. Lie down on the matt and adjust the blanket under you so that you're comfortable.
4. Lay your arms flat on the ground with your palms up, relaxed (your hands can curl naturally). Make sure your neck is in a neutral position (chin pointed towards your chest) and your shoulders are down (not bunched up).
5. Close your eyes and breathe deeply for 10 minutes. You can play meditative music to help you relax.
6. To get out of the position, bend your knees towards your chest, then roll slowly onto your side. When you are ready, lift onto your hands and knees and slowly stand up.

Stretching

Just doing simple stretches will help to release muscular tension, which will in turn, help to reduce stress and induce a state of relaxation. See the stretching exercises in this book as a start. You'll soon discover what relieves the tension in your body by trying a number of different types of stretches.

Massage

Massage releases muscular tension and can be extremely relaxing. Get your partner to give you a massage (returning the favour is relaxing too) or go to a masseuse, and then just lie back and enjoy the occasion.

Acupuncture

This requires a trained specialist who has studied the practice for many years. It can be very effective in inducing a state of relaxation. If you don't like needles, some acupuncturists use pressure points instead.

Tai Chi

Tai Chi is a lovely, gentle exercise that has a meditative component and is excellent for improving balance and coordination. Often practitioners run programs in parks and other open spaces, which makes it particularly pleasant.

Try this simple Tai Chi meditation. It's especially great if you are feeling anxious as it will help you to slow your thinking and control your breathing.

You can do this outside in the sunshine particularly if you need to get away from your desk, for example.

1. Stand with your legs together then step forward with one leg so that it's in front of the other. Your knees should be relaxed. Your feet don't have to be in perfect alignment but they should be pointing forward.
2. Keeping your elbows at waist level, hold your palms out so that they are facing each other. You can also hold a stick between your hands if that helps.
3. Gently rock forward and back in a circular motion, so that your entire upper body is following the movement. Your forward leg should bend to help you balance as you rock.
4. Breathe deeply and if you can, close your eyes to enhance the meditation. Keep on moving and breathing for about 10 minutes.

Hypnosis

Hypnosis is a state of deep relaxation, but it is not something you should do on your own. Find a properly qualified practitioner. Hypnosis has been shown to help with quitting smoking, eating disorders and other problems, so it is worth investigating on a number of levels.

Combining strategies

Louis Proto, the author of *The Alpha Guide to Total Relaxation*, suggests combining a variety of techniques in a five-step relaxation guide. In summary, the process goes like this:

1. Become passive and stop paying attention to the external environment.
2. Repeat a positive mantra silently to yourself, something like 'life is good'.
3. Slow your mind down by deep breathing and counting the breaths.
4. Replace the counting with a calming word, such as 'relax'.
5. Progressively relax all the muscles in your body starting with your toes.

TAKE-HOME MESSAGE

Our lives are stressful. We need to find strategies to manage stress. When you are successful at stress management, you are happier and healthier and better able to withstand the unexpected changes in life. Find a relaxation technique that works for you and practise it.

Conclusion

Putting it all together

In this book I have given you a host of exercise, diet and stress-management tools. It is now up to you to take the information on board and commit to making some changes. The important thing to remember is that small changes can grow into big changes, and even small changes will improve the quality of your life and you will feel better about yourself and the world.

Think about the principles of goal setting and follow the S.M.A.R.T. protocol:

Specific: Make your goals unambiguous; for example, 'I am going to lose 3 centimetres from my waistline' rather than 'I am going to lose weight'.

Measurable: 'I am going to be able to do five push-ups from my knees' rather than 'I would like to do some push-ups'.

Achievable: Wanting to represent Australia in the Olympics is not really achievable for most of us, but we can improve our skills and our fitness. An achievable goal would be something like, 'I'm going to do the full 20 minutes of *LifeSprints*'.

Realistic: This is a bit like achievable goals but deals more with your fantasies. 'I would like to meet a prince and become a princess' is a nice thought but not realistic. And there aren't too many available princes in the world!

Timely: Set a date or timeframe to achieve your goals, such as 'By the end of this month, I am going to stop drinking soft drinks' and then 'I will achieve this by reducing my intake so I have a soft drink every second day, then every third day, and so on, and by the end of the month I will no longer be drinking soft drinks'.

Setting short-term goals that support your ultimate goal/s is the way to make it happen. Perhaps you would like to run a marathon or get back into your size 10 wedding dress (and you are now a size 16). These goals may well seem unattainable and, if so, you may think, 'Why bother?' 'Too hard!' But if you put these ultimate goals on the back burner, and set S.M.A.R.T. short-term goals, you may just reach those long-term goals sooner than you think.

An example of short-term goals (bear in mind, this is *not* a training program for the marathon, it is a goal-setting program) for any would-be marathon runner might be:

I will walk 15 minutes every day this week.
↓
I will walk 30 minutes every day this week.
↓
Every second walk, I will do at least 5 minutes of jogging.
↓
Every second walk, I will do at least 10 minutes of jogging.
↓
Every second walk, I will do at least 20 minutes of jogging.
↓
Every second exercise session, I will jog instead of walk.
↓
I will do a 30-minute jog three times a week.
↓

I will do a 40-minute jog three times a week.

↓

I will do a 50-minute jog three times a week.

↓

I will do a 60-minute jog three times a week and one *LifeSprints* session.

↓

I will do a 1.5-hour jog three times a week and one *LifeSprints* session.

↓

I will do a 1.5-hour jog three times a week and two *LifeSprints* sessions.

↓

I will do a 2-hour jog three times a week and two *LifeSprints* sessions.

↓

I will do a 2.5-hour jog three times a week and two *LifeSprints* sessions.

Before you know it, you are pretty much there!

The trick is, to remember these changes are additive. Make one new change each week, make that change part of your routine and add another new one. And if you want to get back into that wedding dress, your aim might be to lose half a kilogram per week, so you:

- follow the *LifeSprints* training program
- start doing some resistance training
- make short-term goals for dietary change such as, 'This week I will eliminate butter or margarine from my sandwiches' (you'll get used to it quickly).

Small changes you can stick to and build on means that dress is looking good!

Reading list

Below is a selection of scientific papers that provide the evidence for the material in this book. This is not an exhaustive list, but it will give you a chance to read more deeply should it interest you.

Atlantis, E. & Baker, M. (2008), 'Obesity effects on depression: Systematic review of epidemiological studies', *International Journal of Obesity*, 32, 881–91.

Mozaffarian, D., Aruna Kamineni, P.H., Carnethon, M., Djousse, L., Mukamal, K.J. & Siscovick, D. (2009), 'Lifestyle Risk Factors and New-Onset Diabetes Mellitus in Older Adults: The Cardiovascular Health Study', *Archives of Internal Medicine*, 169(8),798–807.

Björntorp, P. (2001), 'Do stress reactions cause abdominal obesity and comorbidities?', *Obesity Reviews*, 2, 73–86.

Popkin, B.M. (2006), 'Global nutrition dynamics: The world is shifting rapidly toward a diet linked with noncommunicable diseases', *American Journal of Clinical Nutrition*, 84, 289–98.

Trapp, E.G., Chisholm, D.J., & Boutcher, S.H. (2007), 'Metabolic response of trained and untrained females during high intensity intermittent cycle exercise', *American Journal of Physiology: Regulatory Integrative and Comparative Physiology*, 293, 2370–5.

Trapp, E.G., Chisholm, D.J., Freund, J., & Boutcher, S.H. (2008), 'The effect of high intensity intermittent exercise training on fat loss and insulin levels of young women', *International Journal of Obesity*, 32(4), 684–91.

Norton, K., Dollman, J., Martin, M. & Harten, N. (2006), 'Descriptive epidemiology of childhood overweight and obesity in Australia: 1901–2003', *International Journal of Pediatric Obesity*, 1, 232–8.

Estruch, R. et al. (2006), 'Effects of a Mediterranean-style diet on cardiovascular risk factors: A randomized trial', *Annals of Internal Medicine*, 145, 1–11.

Shaw, K., Gennat, H., O'Rourke, P. & Del Mar, C. (2006), 'Exercise for overweight or obesity', *Cochrane Database of Systematic Reviews*, Issue 4.

Acknowledgements

Any endeavour such as this is the result of multiple inputs from many people. I would like to thank my colleagues, all the wonderful students at the University of New South Wales who helped in the research leading to this publication and especially the women who worked so hard as subjects in the exercise studies. All the wonderful people at Allen & Unwin have made this possible. Jo Lyons and Bojana Simsic were the gorgeous models for the photographs in the book. My family (husband Geoffrey, daughter Rebecca, son Josef and his wife Tanya, and two very special little characters, Ryan and Amy) deserve a special mention for putting up with me.